Antonio Dal Canton
Teresa Rampino

Lessons of Nephrology

A pocket-size handbook of renal disease

edra

LESSONS OF NEPHROLOGY. A pocket-size handbook of renal disease

Antonio Dal Canton, Teresa Rampino

ISBN: 978-88-214-5329-8
eISBN: 978-88-214-5330-4

Book Publishing Manager: Costanza Smeraldi
Paper, Printing and Binding Manager: Michele Ribatti
Cover: Roberta Venturieri

Layout and Copyediting: ALTER EDOM s.r.l., Noventa Padovana (PD), Italy

Edra S.p.A.
Via G. Spadolini 7, 20141 Milano
Tel. 02 881841

www.edizioniedra.it

Printed in Italy, September 2020

(*) Edra S.p.A. is a part of LSWR GROUP

AUTHORS

Antonio Dal Canton, Former Professor of Nephrology, Università degli Studi di Pavia, Pavia, Italy

Teresa Rampino, Head of Nephrology Dialysis Transplantation Unit, San Matteo Research Hospital, Pavia, Italy

PREFACE

Writing a Nephrology book is not an easy task for anyone. The argument is often difficult, very complicated to explain and it can easily lead to incomprehensibility or even worse to boredom. The question becomes even more complex when one wants to encompass, in few pages, the most salient information, necessary both to understand the complex nature of the kidney and to approach, with appropriate tranquility, a critical patient such as the one with kidney problems.

All this succeeded by prof. Antonio Dal Canton, who in these "Lessons", which are very similar to "Confessions on the Subject", manages to bring out the essentials of Nephrology, without falling into banality and above all without boring. The whole book, and in particular the chapters dedicated to Water, Eelectrolytes and Acid-Base Disorders, can be read with pleasure, thanks to a fluent and sometimes even lovable lexicon, embellished in several points by these "Curious Questions" that make it alive, practical and never tiring.

Curiosity, which is one of the greatest merits of the expert researcher, has always accompanied the professional life of Professor Dal Canton. This merit combined with his great passion for the study of the Greek-Latin world (to underline the continuous references to the etymology of the medical lexicon) were the ideal prerequisites for creating a small masterpiece of International Nephrological Literature. Finally, all the chapters show his extraordinary ability to "teach" Nephrological Science to students and young doctors, a further constant feature of his long and prestigious academic career.

Antonio considers himself to be an excellent sailor and often likes to repeat that he willingly accepts criticism of his professional skills, but not to bear any notes on his being a "Sea Dog".

I believe that his journey into the world of Nephrology is at least equal to one of his adventurous crossings of the *Mare Nostrum*.

Giovambattista Capasso
Full Professor of Nephrology
Director of Department of Translational Medical Sciences
Università degli studi della Campania Luigi Vanvitelli
President of Italian Board of Nephrology Professors

ACKNOWLEDGMENTS

I would like to thank professor Vittorio E. Andreucci for having read the manuscript with the spirit of a peer reviewer, spending so much time and providing comments and suggestions as only an outstanding scientist and educator as he is could do.

I would also like to address special thanks to the thousands of students that I had the privilege to meet during my 40 years teaching in five different universities. They have been an invaluable source of curiosity and color throughout my life. I appreciate them all.

Prof. Antonio Dal Canton

ABBREVIATIONS

AA	amyloid A
ACE	angiotensin-converting enzyme
ADH	antidiuretic hormone
AG	anion gap
AII	angiotensin II
AKI	acute kidney injury
AL	amyloid light-chain
ANCA	anti-neutrophil cytoplasmic antibody
APD	automated peritoneal dialysis
ARF	acute renal failure
ATN	acute tubular necrosis
ATPase	adenosinetriphosphatase
AVF	arteriovenous fistula
BP	blood pressure
BUN	blood urea nitrogen
BW	body weight
CAPD	continuous ambulatory peritoneal dialysis
CMV	cytomegalovirus
CRD	chronic renal disease
CRF	chronic renal failure
CT	computed tomography
CVC	central venous catheter
DBD	donor after brain death
DCD	donor after circulatory death
DGF	delayed graft function
DIC	disseminated intravascular coagulation
EBV	effective blood volume
ECF	extracellular fluid
ECG	electrocardiogram
EPH	edema, proteinuria, hypertension
EPO	erythropoietin
FENa	fractional excretion of filtered sodium
FGF23	fibroblast growth factor 23
GBM	glomerular basement membrane
GFR	glomerular filtration rate

HD	hemodialysis
HE	hematoxylin/eosin
HELLP	hemolysis elevated liver enzymes low platelet
HIP	hypertension in pregnancy
HIV	human immunodeficiency virus
HLA	human leucocyte antigen
HSP	Henoch-Schönlein purpura
HUS	hemolytic uremic syndrome
IC	immune complexes
ICF	intracellular fluid
ICU	intensive care unit
IgA	immunoglobulin A
IU	international unit
LCDD	light-chain deposition disease
LDH	lactate dehydrogenase
MCD	medullary cystic disease
MHC	major histocompatibility complex
NPT	nephronophthisis
PD	peritoneal dialysis
PEG	percutaneous endoscopic gastrostomy
PIH	pregnancy induced hypertension
PKD	polycystic kidney disease
PTH	parathyroid hormone
RAS	renin-angiotensin system
ROS	reactive oxygen species
RRT	renal replacement therapy
SAA	serum amyloid A
SGA	small for gestational age
SIADH	syndrome of inappropriate ADH secretion
SLE	systemic lupus erythematosus
TBC	tuberculosis
TM	thrombotic microangiopathy
TPR	total peripheral resistance
UTI	urinary tract infection
VEGF	vascular endothelial growth factor
VEGFR	vascular endothelial growth factor receptor
vWF	von Willebrand factor

CONTENTS

SECTION 5

THE KIDNEY IN PREGNANCY

SECTION 6

DEGENERATIVE AND HEREDITARY RENAL DISORDERS

APPENDICES

SECTION 1

DISORDERS OF BODY FLUID VOLUME AND ELECTROLYTE COMPOSITION

CHAPTER 1

DISORDERS OF EXTRACELLULAR FLUID VOLUME

As tough as it may seem, the human body is made mainly with water. The fraction that is represented by water ranges from 60% to 70% and depends on age, sex and body fat amount. Children are more "watery" than adults, and body water decreases in the elderly. Females have more fat and less water than males but pregnancy is a very unique condition in which extracellular fluid volume increases by 15% (see Chapter 11).

Two thirds of body water are inside the cells (Intracellular Fluid, ICF), one third is outside of the cells (Extracellular Fluid, ECF). In turn, ECF is distributed in different compartments. Its major fraction is in the interstice, and most of the remaining part is inside the circulatory system. Small volumes of ECF are contained in joints (synovial fluid), brain (liquor), and eye. In pathological conditions ECF accumulates in the pleural or peritoneal cavity and in the pericardium.

The most "important" part of ECF is that contained in the circulation, on which depends the delivery of nutrients and oxygen to peripheral tissues. Indeed, the systems that regulate ECF volume utilize blood volume both as the index of ECF status and as the target of regulation. One important concept is that the volume of blood perceived by the regulatory systems is not the total volume of blood that is contained in vessels, but the volume of blood that is actually circulating (Effective Blood Volume, EBV). The difference between total blood volume and EBV is accounted for by the "capacitance vessels", i.e. the venous vessels that behave like an elastic tank that expands and collapses thereby changing the blood that is distributed to the peripheral tissue.

BODY SODIUM CONTENT IS THE DETERMINANT OF ECF VOLUME

All cells have in their plasma membrane the Na^+/K^+ adenosine triphosphatase (ATPase) pump that drives sodium out and potassium into the cell. The sodium concentration gradient generated by the pump is steep, approximately 140 (out) vs. 10 (in) mmol/L, and characterizes the ECF as a "sodium space". Sodium is present in body water in ion form and its cumulative electric positive charge is neutralized by an equivalent mass of anions, the main ones being chloride and bicarbonate.

In view of the almost total distribution of sodium in the extracellular space the osmotic attraction generated by sodium retains water out of the cells and the more sodium is present in the body, the more expanded is its ECF volume. Normal sodium concentration averages 140 mmol/L (range 135-145 mmol/L), so that in clinical practice it can be assumed that the addition of 140 mmol of sodium to body sodium mass expands ECF volume by 1 L and the opposite holds for the loss of 140 mmol.

It must be stressed that ECF volume depends on the content, i.e. the mass of sodium present in the body, that is expressed in weight units. The mass of sodium must not be confused with serum sodium concentration that is expressed in weight/volume units. Misunderstanding mass for concentration is a gross mistake and the difference between the two concepts seems obvious, but in clinical practice the distinction is often obscured by tricky circumstances that deviate rational thinking to wrong conclusions.

ESTIMATE OF ECF VOLUME IN CLINICAL PRACTICE

A pathological depletion/expansion of ECF volume is one of the most common clinical problems met in daily practice. Unfortunately, there is no laboratory, radiological, or instrumental way to measure ECF volume and understanding its state rests on clinical experience and physical examination. Observing the patient for some consecutive days is often the clue to understand the dynamics of ECF volume. In particular a very simple way to detect changes in body fluid is to weigh regularly the patient, assuming that in the short term of a few days weight changes of 0.5 kg or more are not caused by fat or muscle mass variation.

SIGNS OF DEPLETION

Blood pressure (BP) measured in the supine position and soon after the patient stood up is a way to check volume depletion, that is suggested by a decrease in diastolic blood pressure. A decline of 3 or more mm Hg is considered in some textbooks as diagnostic. But at least 5 mm Hg are realistic, considering the confounding factors that are associated with the maneuver. The test is biased by conditions that block the reflex vasoconstriction such as autonomic nervous insufficiency or antihypertensive drugs.

Normally in a subject laying supine jugular vein is visible up to the mandibular angle, finding it collapsed at a lower level indicates volume depletion.

Additional physical findings suggesting volume depletion involve the tongue and skin. The tongue may show transversal furrows and may appear dry; sometimes, however, the tongue is dry because the patient is breathing with the mouth open; in these cases it should be checked whether the oral mucosa is dry under the tongue. The skin may have lost its elasticity, which can be detected by pinching it to form a fold and observing how fast it flattens.

Thirst is a subjective sign of volume depletion, that depends on stimulation of brain thirst centers by angiotensin II, produced by activation of the renin-angiotensin system (RAS). On evaluating thirst as indicator of volume depletion the alternative possibility of a rise in plasma osmolality has to be considered.

A rise in hematocrit and serum protein concentration detected by serial measurements in a time of some days indicates volume depletion. Note that hematocrit does not change when the loss of fluid is limited to pure water because water is lost in the same proportion from the intra- and extracellular volume, so that the ratio of red blood cell volume over plasma volume remains the same.

Finally, volume depletion activates humoral, hemodynamic and nervous signals that reduce renal sodium excretion (in a urine sample the sodium concentration will be low), mainly by increasing tubular sodium reabsorption. This sign, however, must be interpreted in single cases because urinary sodium retention can be the response to a decrease in EBV, that does not depend on sodium depletion, but is rather associated with excess ECF volume, e.g. congestive heart failure (see later).

SIGNS OF EXPANSION

Peripheral edema, i.e. swelling due to accumulation of fluid in the interstice, is the paradigm of ECF excess. Usually edema is localized in the legs where fluid is drained by gravity, but in bedridden people it distributes throughout the lower part of the body and it is particularly visible in the sacral region. A popular diagnostic maneuver consists of pressing fingers on the tibial plate and observing the formation of a deep pit. A common mistake made by beginners checking for pitting edema is to press the leg too lightly to displace interstitial fluid.

Pitting edema indicates a fluid retention of around 5 kg in a 70 kg body weight person.

Hypertension, dilution of hematocrit and serum protein concentration are accessory signs of expansion, but they are affordable only if their change is documented in a quick follow up after a few days.

Excess ECF can accumulate in the lung, usually as pleural effusion or in the tissue. In the latter case, rales can be detected by auscultation, but sometimes the fluid is interstitial and physical examination fails to detect it, a case that is particularly frequent in uremic patients.

Causes of ECF volume depletion

Gastrointestinal disorders that cause diarrhea or vomiting and stop or reduce eating and drinking are the most frequent cause of ECF volume depletion. Diuretics are common culprits, usually when their assumption is continued in a condition in which feeding and drinking ability is decreased, e.g. in patients with low consciousness or elderly subjects in rest homes.

Skin is a source of fluid loss, either as *perspiratio insensibilis* or as sweat. Note that sweating and *perspiratio insensibilis*, however, contain a low sodium amount (sweat) or no sodium at all (*perspiratio insensibilis*), therefore they cause a loss of water rather than of sodium and have the major effect on plasma osmolality (see later). However, profuse sweating may cause severe ECF volume depletion.

Also burns and severe inflammatory disease of the skin cause loss of fluid with protein concentration similar to that of plasma with a dramatic effect on plasma volume.

"Salt-losing nephropathies" are renal disorders that decrease the tubular ability to reabsorb sodium such as chronic pyelonephritis and adult polycystic kidney disease.

Pressure diuresis is an experimental natriuresis caused by a steep rise in renal arterial perfusion pressure. It occurs when perfusion pressure rises beyond the limit of renal autoregulation. Renal autoregulation is the phenomenon by which renal blood flow and the glomerular filtration rate (GFR) remain constant at variations of perfusion pressure between 180 and 80 mm Hg.

"Exaggerated natriuresis" consists of the very prompt and massive elimination of an intravenous sodium load that occurs in hypertensive patients. The phenomenon depends on renal vasodilation induced by ECF volume expansion that blocks the vasoconstrictive response of autoregulation. On their own, "pressure natriuresis" and "exaggerated natriuresis" are experimental models that do not reproduce clinical conditions. However, they are a clue to understanding the mechanisms that account for renal sodium loss in malignant hypertension and hypertension in pregnancy (see Chapter 11).

Hypercalcemia, especially when associated with malignancy, affects sodium reabsorption by inhibiting tubular Na/K exchanger an Na/H cotransporter, and can induce massive saline diuresis.

Major surgery, especially when requiring laparotomy, is at risk for volume depletion, because of the loss of blood, drying of peritoneal surface, wound leakage, post-surgery bowel palsy with luminal fluid sequestration, and post-surgery fasting. The amount of fluid that is lost in this setting is often underestimated and the infusion program is often not adequate to maintain or recover fluid balance, a failure that can depend on the method by which patient fluid need is calculated (see later).

Causes of ECF volume expansion

Two distinct pathogenic mechanisms can account for sodium and water retention, one resulting from the response of functioning kidneys to deceiving information on body sodium content, the other one dependent on kidney failure.

It is intriguing that in most cases peripheral edema occurs because the kidneys comply correctly with an incorrect order. In fact, the salt retaining sequence is turned on by a defect of EBV that is perceived by regulatory systems as a loss of ECF volume, i.e. of body sodium mass. The kidney is forced to recover sodium that does not improve EBV but accumulates out of the circulation.

The most common condition of peripheral edema is congestive heart failure. In the past, two pathogenic mechanisms were in competition to explain fluid retention in heart failure, the so-called "anterograde" and "retrograde" theories. The former pointed to low cardiac output that evoked renal avidity for sodium. The retrograde theory pointed to the difficulty of the failing heart to receive blood preload and to the consequent rise in venous pressure transmitted to the peripheral capillary circulation. Here, the rise in hydrostatic pressure prevails over oncotic pressure and the imbalance between the two Starling forces shifts fluid in the interstice.

The simple consideration that the amount of fluid that generates a pitting edema is about 5 L, and that the total volume of plasma is about 2-3 L, makes the retrograde theory unrealistic.

What really occurs is that fluid is retained by the kidney to restore circulating blood volume, but the kidney's effort cannot be successful because the problem is pump failure, not lack of fluid.

Low EBV is the pathogenic mechanism of edema also in nephrotic syndrome. Nephrotic syndrome is a cluster of symptoms that are edema, high grade proteinuria (>3 g/24 h), low plasma protein with altered protein fractions, and hypercholesterolemia. The symptoms start with proteinuria. Note that proteinuria indicates an abnormal permeability of glomerular capillaries that can be caused by diverse diseases with different pathogenic mechanisms (see Chapter 5). Protein loss is followed by a decrease in plasma protein concentration with a prevalent effect on low molecular weight albumin. The albumin fraction of plasma proteins falls below 50% while large proteins, namely alpha-2 globulins rise from about 10-12% up to 30%.

As part of its response to protein loss the liver increases protein synthesis including lipoproteins that, like alpha-2 globulin, are big and accumulate in serum where they bind lipids, increasing circulating lipid levels. Formation of edema starts with the imbalance of Starling forces due to low oncotic pressure that shifts fluid from the intravascular compartment to the interstice. The ensuing hypovolemia triggers sodium retention through neural, hemodynamic and humoral effectors. A main effector is the renin-angiotensin system that is strongly activated and stimulates aldosterone release. In fact, aldosterone was discovered in a patient with nephrotic syndrome in which plasma levels of aldosterone were so high as to be detectable with the rudimentary biochemistry means available in the 1930s.

Liver cirrhosis is associated with fluid retention that mostly accumulates as ascites, but in a minority of patients also causes peripheral edema. Ascites results from increased pressure in the portal circulation and low serum albumin. Both of these phenomena contribute to generate an imbalance in Starling forces and the prevalence of hydrostatic over oncotic pressure moves fluid out of the capillary.

Quite surprisingly, chronic renal failure is not as frequently the cause of peripheral edema. In fact, in chronic renal failure the decrease in the amount of filtered sodium causes sodium retention, but to a limited extent because ECF volume and effective blood volume rise proportionally and hypervolemia inhibits tubular sodium reabsorption. Also in acute renal failure oliguria is rarely associated with edema. In cases treated with dialysis fluid is removed by ultrafiltration (see Chapter 9), while in patients on conservative treatment, restriction of salt is often sufficient to limit ECF volume expansion till GFR is recovered.

HOW TO TREAT DISORDERS OF ECF VOLUME

The disorders of ECF volume are treated as disorders of sodium mass, i.e. by adding sodium to the body or subtracting it, in cases of ECF volume depletion or expansion, respectively. Sodium is delivered orally or intravenously, as sodium chloride or sodium bicarbonate. We do not recommend solutions of sodium lactate or citrate that are available as substitutes for bicarbonate, because they need metabolic transformation to generate bicarbonate and the rate of the metabolic process is not predictable. Their use can be advantageous in patients that need calcium because calcium can be mixed with them remaining soluble, while it precipitates as carbonate in a bicarbonate solution.

Sodium chloride has a molecular weight of 58 daltons, and 1 g delivers 17 mmol of sodium, while sodium bicarbonate weights 84 daltons and 1 g delivers 12 mmol of sodium.

Excess ECF volume is treated by reducing dietary sodium intake or by using diuretics. In fact, currently used diuretics are natriuretic drugs, that reduce tubular sodium reabsorption and drag water to urine by osmotic drive. Diuretic drugs that are currently used are thiazides (chlortalidone and hydrochlorothiazide) and high-ceiling diuretics (furosemide, ethacrynic acid, bumetanide). The first ones inhibit sodium reabsorption in the early tract of distal tubule, the

(iii) Sum the loss of water, sodium, potassium from all sources but urine. Distinguish the fraction of sodium lost as chloride or bicarbonate.

(iv) Add to the losses calculated in (iii) the amount of water and electrolytes that you wish to eliminate in the urine (urinary sodium is eliminated as chloride). The resulting sum is the amount of water and electrolyte to be delivered during the next 24 h, timing the sequence and rate of infusion of different solutions with a priority determined by clinical risk, e.g. consider whether to address first a volume or a pH problem.

(v) Twenty-four hours after the start of IV infusion program compare the amount of water and electrolytes eliminated in urine with that wished by you as your target. The difference estimates your precision in evaluating losses. Correct the infusion program and repeat the procedure until the amounts (actual and programmed) coincide.

Patient with renal failure

In the patient with renal failure the kidney is not able to adjust water and electrolyte excretion and attain water and electrolyte balance obviating the gap between actual and calculated losses. The diagnosis of body fluid disorders is based on history, evaluation of losses, physical examination and plasma electrolyte concentration. From the information thus obtained state if ECF volume is depleted, normal or expanded. Now calculate an infusion program that includes urine in losses. Monitoring is essential to be prompt in modulating fluid therapy. Careful recording of body weight, blood pressure and urine volume and physical examination, in particular lung and heart auscultation are essential support to decision making. Avoid contradictions or misunderstanding, e.g. do not deliver a saline load associated with diuretic drugs. The two treatments conflict, one increasing sodium gain the other one increasing sodium loss. One of the two treatments is obviously wrong, but the mistake is much more common than expected mainly when protocol infusions are not cross-checked vs. individual prescriptions.

A major mistake is misinterpreting natremia (i.e. the serum concentration of sodium. Sodium symbol is Na from the Latin *natrium*) as an indicator of sodium content in the body, i.e. of ECF volume. In fact, natremia is an indicator of plasma osmolality.

Note: in general the combined administration of saline and diuretics makes no sense. Exceptions are rare, for example to increase urinary calcium excretion in cases of severe hypercalcemia.

CHAPTER 2

DISORDERS OF PLASMA OSMOLALITY AND ICF VOLUME

The kidney regulates plasma osmolality adjusting the amount of water excreted. Renal handling of water is one of the most fascinating achievements of evolution: oversimplifying the process, in the thick tract sodium is pumped out of the lumen leaving water inside because this part of tubule is water-impermeable.

Thus, tubular fluid running out of the loop is hypotonic (30 mOsm/kg). Sodium pumped in interstice increases local sodium concentration and generates a gradient that drives sodium into the adjacient tract of descending limb. Thus, fluid flowing down to the medulla is hypertonic. Multiplication of this process as the hairpin loop deepens into the medulla increases progressively interstitial and luminal sodium concentration and osmolality to a maximum at the tip of 1,200 mOsm/kg.Thus the countercurrent mechanism generates a steep corticomedullary osmotic gradient that permits a fine modulation of final urine concentration. In fact, the permeability to water of collecting ducts is regulated by ADH (pitressin) so that the higher ADH levels the higher permeability, osmotic reabsorption of water from luminal fluid and final urine concentration.

In turn, ADH is the effector of two systems that regulate its secretion, one that finely regulates ADH release according to plasma osmolality, the other one quite grossly dependent on EBV. As will be discussed later, the second mechanism is not as important in the physiological regulation of water balance, but it has a main pathogenic role in common disorders associated with hyponatremia. In any case, it is important to understand that the kidney regulates plasma osmolality by changing water not solute excretion, therefore disorders of plasma osmolality are disorders of water metabolism.

Any addition/loss of water to/from the body distributes in ICF and ECF in proportion with the part of total body fluid they represent, i.e. 2/3 and 1/3 respectively. Any change in body water content impacts on the volume and osmolality of both the compartments, but the changes of ICV have dramatic effects on cell volume, shape and structure, that jeopardize important cell functions.

In conclusion: when we think of a problem dealing with body fluid osmolality, we have to handle the problem as a matter of water. Osmolality of body fluids impacts on cell volume, it is the determinant of ICF volume.

NATREMIA: AN INDEX OF PLASMA OSMOLALITY

Sodium is the most exclusive ion of ECF. Its plasma concentration averages 140 mEq/L. Furthermore its positive electric charge recruits equivalent negative charges, so that sodium and its accompanying anions account for 280 mEq (mOsm)/L, i.e. almost all of the normal plasma osmolality, that averages 300 mOsm/L. Therefore, in clinical practice plasma sodium concentration is currently used as a substitute for plasma osmolality.

There are two exceptions in which natremia does not represent a valuable index of plasma osmolality: hyperglycemia and pseudo-hyponatremia. In type 2 diabetes, hyperglycemia can cause hyperosmolar coma, but natremia is low because glucose attracts water out of the cells causing hemodilution.

As for pseudohyponatremia, it is quite a rare condition in which plasma levels of lipid or protein, i.e. two components that are not soluble in water, are strikingly high as it can occur in inherited hypertriglyceridemia or myeloma. Consider, for example, that triglyceride levels are so high as to represent 10% of plasma volume. This fraction does not contain water nor sodium so that the amount of sodium per unit plasma volume is reduced by 10%. Actually, sodium concentration in plasma water, that is the determinant of osmotic effects, is not reduced, and hyponatremia is "false" (false is the meaning of the Greek word *pseudo*).

HYPONATREMIA

Hyponatremia: with ECF expansion

The most frequent conditions in which hyponatremia occurs are the common causes of peripheral edema. In fact, in congestive heart failure, nephrotic syndrome and liver cirrhosis edema and hyponatremia share the same pathogenic mechanism, i.e. a low EBV that, on the one hand stimulates renal reabsorption of sodium and water and on the other hand raises ADH release and reabsorption of free water. These combined effects of EBV deficiency result in excess salt and water in the body with a disproportionate retention of water. Salt load generates peripheral edema, water excess is responsible for hyponatremia

Inappropriate ADH secretion is a cause of hyponatremia that is associated with solid tumors, lung inflammatory disease, and

CURIOUS QUESTION

Evolution multifunction models

The countercurrent multiplication system is the genial invention of evolution that permits the regulating of urine water excretion. Evolution has used the same invention for a different function. What function in what animal?

Answer: penguins have developed a foot-heating system based on countercurrent multiplication. Without the heater penguin feet would freeze, especially while they are hatching and stand immobile for days.

drug side effects. It depends on the release of ADH or ADH-similar products by cells in the tumor or in inflamed tissue. The condition has to be distinguished from excess water drinking (polydipsia), a compulsive psychiatric disorder. Differential diagnosis rests on the response to a thirst test. Water deprivation is followed by a prompt increase in urine osmolality and a rise in natremia in polydipsia.

It may be unexpected to the reader that the kidney with chronic renal disease maintains the ability to produce free water down to GFR as low as 20 mL/min. Actually, free water clearance[1] and GFR decrease proportionally, so that fractional free water clearance (free water clearance/GFR) is conserved and in most patients it fulfills the task of osmotic regulation in routine daily life. Retention of water is a major risk in patients with very low GFR and in patients on regular dialysis treatment (see Chapter 9).

A special condition of physiological hyponatremia is normal pregnancy in which the feedback regulation of ADH release works perfectly but is reset to a lower level of natremia for a given ADH level.

Hyponatremia: with normal or depleted ECF volume

The most common cause of hyponatremia with depleted ECF is diuretic treatment. Actually diuretics by themselves increase both sodium and water excretion to a similar extent and hyponatremia results from "inappropriate" ADH secretion and from the increase of water drinking. Although in normal conditions ADH secretion depends mainly on the serum osmolality, in severe salt depletion with marked contraction of ECF volume, the main stimulus for ADH secretion becomes the condition of hypovolemia. In these circumstances the need for correcting the hypovolemia is prevailing on the maintenance of normal osmolality by ADH. The water drinking is caused by thirst

1 Free water clearance (C_{H_2O}) is calculated as the difference of urinary volume (V) less osmolar clearance (C_{OSM}). It is positive when urine osmolality (U_{OSM}) is lower than plasma osmolality (P_{OSM}). When urine osmolality is higher than plasma osmolality free water clearance is negative (it measures the volume of blood that is completely cleaned of osmoles) and it is symbolized T^cH_2O.

CURIOUS QUESTION

Sophisticated reagents: store at −4° C

Robert, a 55 years old man, has asked his doctor for a visit, because his legs are swollen.

"Did you note whether your urine is foamy?" asks the doctor after visiting Robert.

"Yes, it is! Why do you suspect that?" Robert says, quite surprised.

"You can understand the reason why your urine is foamy by taking something out of your fridge... putting it in a glass of water and shaking" replies the doctor.

What is there in the fridge that can make water foamy?

Answer: the doctor believes that Robert has a nephrotic syndrome and eliminates an abundant amount of protein in urine, mostly represented by albumin. Albumin is a powerful surfactant. The name albumin comes from Latin *albus* that means white. *Albumen* is the Latin name of the white of an egg, that is rich in albumin. The foamy aspect of urine can be reproduced by shaking the white of an egg in water.

stimulated by ECF volume depletion. In particular, thirst is induced by angiotensin II, the effector of the renin-angiotensin system, that stimulates the brain thirst center.

As mentioned above, hyperglycemia causes hyponatremia by extracting water out of the intracellular compartment. Water dilutes all extracellular blood components including electrolytes. Indeed, this is a case in which hyponatremia is not an index of low plasma osmolality, that is actually high due to glucose load. Mannitol, administered to treat post-insult brain edema behaves similarly as hyperglycemia.

Moderate hyponatremia occurs in endocrine disorders, e.g. adrenal insufficiency (Addison's disease) and in hypothyroidism. In the former, the mechanism is related with ECF volume depletion secondary to mineralocorticoid defect and the ensuing stimulation of ADH secretion. In the latter the pathogenesis is less clear, but it does not seem to be ADH-dependent. Rather, it may be related with reduced glomerular filtration rate and decreased sodium delivery to diluting segment (see chapter on potassium disorders).

Symptoms and treatment of hyponatremia

Symptoms of hyponatremia are neurologic. They usually start with nausea, headache and confusion and progress to a widely variable constellation that includes lethargy, seizures, posture instability and lastly coma. The symptoms usually appear at levels of 110-115 mEq/L, but their severity depends mainly on the rapidity of onset.

Treatment aims to correct the imbalance between water and sodium content in the body and priority must be given to the elimination of water rather than the introduction of sodium. This is mandatory in patients with severe ECF volume expansion such as patients with congestive heart failure, in which salt addition to the existing overload can be lethal. Unfortunately, the only available drug that can induce a pure water diuresis is the competitive inhibitor of ADH tolvaptan (a vasopressin type 2 receptor antagonist that is also called acquaretic), that up to now has been licensed by Food and Drug Administration (FDA) and European Medicines Agency (EMA) only for the syndrome of inappropriate ADH (SIADH) secretion. Therefore, water restriction is the only way to reduce body water without also manipulating sodium balance. In the clinical settings of peripheral edema, diuretics used to induce sodium loss have an unpredictable effect on natremia, because of the counteracting effects on free water generation, sodium delivery

CURIOUS QUESTION

Why did you never think of this question: Do fishes drink?

(It means whether they drink by intention, not whether they exchange water through the skin.)

Answer: salt water fishes do drink, fresh water fishes do not. Why? The salt concentration in sea water is higher than in blood, so that salt water fishes lose water through the skin. They must recover water but the only water available is sea water that would further increase plasma osmolality. Nevertheless, they drink salt water, but eliminate excess salt through a special sodium excreting gland located in the gills. Fresh water fishes have the opposite problem, i.e. they absorb excess water through the skin so that drinking would further dilute their blood. They do not drink and eliminate excess water in urine, thanks to a powerful diluting capacity of the kidney.

to the diluting segment, and ADH release after volume depletion. In fact thiazides inhibit sodium reabsorption in diluting segment and reduce free water generation while furosemide increases the amount of sodium that is delivered to the diluting segment, and increases free water generation. Furthermore, both thiazides and furosemide deplete ECF volume and stimulate volume-dependent ADH release.

Inducing sweating is a rationale way to cause a loss of water exceeding the loss of salt, but the results are not predictable, not only because of the intrinsic difficulty in quantifying sweat loss, but also because sweat sodium concentration varies in a wide range, from 40 to 80 mEq/L.

Infusion of hypertonic saline solution is indicated only in symptomatic patients with severe hyponatremia (<130 mEq/L). Caution is necessary when infusing salt, because it expands ECF volume increasing the risk of acute cardiovascular failure. Prevention of such an ominous complication as pulmonary edema by coadministration of diuretic is mandatory in cardiac patients. Hypertonic saline infusion is the straightforward treatment of hyponatremia associated with ECF volume depletion, a condition in which sodium loading is indicated not only to increase natremia, but to expand ECF.

In any case, the infusion of hypertonic saline must be slow, aiming at increasing sodium concentration at a rate lower than 6 mEq/24 h in order to prevent the dramatic complication of pontine myelinolysis, neurologic disorder that causes cognitive and movement symptoms. Rarely, the latter consist of a paralysis that involves all but the eye muscles (so called "locked-in syndrome").

HYPERNATREMIA

Hypernatremia occurs usually as the consequence of loss of water either alone or together with a lower amount of sodium and in most cases is associated with depletion of ECF.

Hypernatremia with ECF volume depletion

Cerebral breathing in patients with acute brain injury is a paradigm of pure water loss. In fact, the high rate and increased depth of open-mouthed breathing dissipates liters of water in a day.

Sweat is hypotonic, so that abundant sweating per se causes dehydration and volume depletion. In people with preserved thirst to whom water is available, drinking compensates for the loss of water and can even turn the effect of sweating from a risk of hypernatremia to an actual hyponatremia.

The elderly, especially those with dementia or advanced Parkinson's disease that are unable or unwilling to take oral feeding are at risk of dehydration. In particular, in subjects on enteral tube feeding the need for water can change, depending on environmental factors, such as temperature and humidity as well as personal circumstances, e.g. fever. In these people the negative water balance is usually associated with ECF moderate volume depletion. The associated cognitive deficiency masks neurological symptoms, therefore natremia should be regularly monitored.

Hypernatremia with ECF volume expansion

The most frequent setting in which hypernatremia is associated with volume expansion is iatrogenic and consists of a patient that can not drink and is infused with hypertonic saline. Poor drinking is the necessary premise that accounts for hypernatremia in patients with primary hyperaldosteronism and corticosteroid treatment.

Symptoms and treatment of hypernatremia

Symptoms of hypernatremia are neurological and are similar to those of hyponatremia, i.e. they consist of lethargy, muscle cramps, nausea, headache, seizures and coma. Water is the treatment and in many cases it has to be delivered by intravenous route as isotonic (5%) glucose solution. In fact, IV infusion of pure water cannot be done because it would cause hemolysis; on the other hand, the presence of glucose does not compromise the hydration of the patient since glucose is rapidly consumed by normal metabolism.

Insulin can be added if necessary, e.g. in diabetic patients, one IU every 4 g of glucose. The infusion of glucose solution has to be slow, having as target a change in sodium concentration lower than 5.0 mMol/day. Higher rates can determine cerebral edema.

TRICKY CASE? N. 1

An 80 year old woman is admitted to hospital with lateral left palsy, cerebral breathing, severe hypertension. Brain CT scan shows parietal right hemorrhage. Blood biochemistry shows hypernatremia (158 mMol/L), high BUN (70 mg/dL), high serum creatinine (3.2 mg/dL).

"Sodium is very high" says the doctor on call to the nurse.
"And she has an advanced renal failure. A large amount of furosemide will be necessary to eliminate excess sodium" the sister comments.

Here are two possible responses of the doctor:

ANSWER 1
"Right! Prepare furosemide 100 mg, intravenously."

ANSWER 2
"She doesn't need diuretic."

Which of the two responses is correct?

Disclosure: response 2 is correct.
In this patient hypernatremia indicates water loss caused by hyperventilation. Brain injury made it impossible to introduce water and food and probably also her sodium balance was negative, Thus, she had a deficit of water and sodium but the deficit of water was greater. Hence the rise in plasma osmolality, that is treated by giving water rather than by increasing sodium excretion. Diuretic would increase sodium excretion and worsen ECF volume depletion.

CHAPTER 3

DISORDERS OF BODY FLUID POTASSIUM

Potassium is the prevalent ion of intracellular fluid and, according to the Nernst equation[2], it is the determinant of transmembrane electrical potential.

The message of the equation is that transmembrane potassium concentration gradient is the determinant of cell membrane potential. In the resting condition cells are polarized with the negative pole inside cell.

The potential difference is −90 mVolt. An increase in potassium concentration out of the cell, according to the Nernst equation ($\log K_o - \log K_i$) makes potential differences less negative, i.e. depolarizes cell membrane that becomes more excitable. Thus, changes in serum potassium affect cell excitability, increasing the risk for conduction disorders, in particular cardiac arrhythmia and arrest.

---

2 Nernst equation: $E = RT/G \times \log K_o/K_i = RT/G \times (\log K_o - \log k_i)$.
Where: E is the transmembrane electric potential at rest, RT/G is a constant, $\log K_o/K_i$ is the natural logarithm of fraction extracellular/ over intracellular potassium concentration. Logarithm of a fraction in mathematics corresponds to the difference of numerator log less denominator log.

DETERMINANTS OF SERUM POTASSIUM CONCENTRATION

Normal serum potassium concentration ranges from 3.5 to 5.0 mMol/L and is regulated by the kidney that adapts its excretion to the variable amount introduced with food. In the kidney potassium is freely filtered and then reabsorbed almost completely in the proximal tubule. Urinary potassium comes from the distal part of the nephron where the principal cells reabsorb sodium exchanging it for potassium. Therefore, potassium excretion is strictly dependent on the two main determinants of sodium reabsorption by principal cells, i.e. aldosterone and distal sodium delivery.

As for the mechanisms by which aldosterone and distal delivery regulate sodium reabsorption, aldosterone binds to intranuclear receptors generating a signal that is transduced into enhanced number of Na^+/K^+ exchangers expressed in the basolateral membrane. The effect of the delivery depends on the phenomenon by which, for a given level of aldosterone the activity of the principal cells is grossly proportional to the amount of sodium that escapes reabsorption in the proximal part of the nephron. Actually, principal cells behave like employees paid for piecework, i.e. the more work is committed to them, the more work they do. A further factor that modulates potassium excretion is blood pH. In fact, acidemia shifts potassium out of the cells, decreases intracellular potassium concentration and lowers the gradient between ICF and ECF, while alkalemia has the opposite effect. This pH dependent redistribution of K ions occurs also in principal cells and contrasts potassium excretion by decreasing gradient between intracellular and luminal potassium concentration and gradient-dependent excretory drive.

HYPERKALEMIA

Hyperkalemia is a major cause of death in patients with acute renal failure (ARF), especially in those that are oliguric. Actually, in ARF potassium retention, metabolic acidosis and often release of potassium from cell lysis concur to generate very severe hyperkalemia, topping in our experience at 9.4 mEq/L (the patient survived!).

Hyperkalemia is also a common finding in patients with chronic renal disease and GFR <30 mL/min, but usually it is moderate as long as renal function approaches the need for renal replacement treatment (see Chapter 9). In patients with chronic renal disease, severe hyperkalemia can occur as the side effects of drugs that inhibit the activity of Na^+/K^+ tubular exchange, in particular drugs that reduce aldosterone levels, i.e. ACE inhibitors and angiotensin II antagonists, or compete for nuclear aldosterone receptor (spironolactone), or block potassium channels such as triamterene and amiloride, the so-called potassium sparing diuretics.

Serum potassium can also increase in patients with normal renal function after the release of a massive potassium load from cell lysis, e.g. hemolysis, rhabdomyolysis, chemotherapy of lymphoma, gastrointestinal hemorrhage.

Hyperkalemia is part of the symptoms of renal tubular acidosis type 4 or generalized distal tubular acidosis. The pathogenic mechanism consists of a failure of mineralocorticoid activity in the distal tubule, that can be caused by a wide variety of genetic or acquired defects. Blocking aldosterone hampers both potassium excretion and proton expulsion by intercalated cells.

Symptoms and treatment of hyperkalemia

Skeletal muscle weakness up to flaccid paralysis and cardiac arrhythmias including bradyarrhythmia, ventricular fibrillation up to asystole are the symptoms of hyperkalemia. Muscle block can be misdiagnosed as a neurological problem. Often, ECG changes are the first clue to diagnosis. The ECG changes consist of the flattening of P wave, enlargement of the QRS complex and of T wave. In severe cases monster QRS and T disproportionately high and large are barely identifiable as recordings of ventricular electric activity.

Hyperkalemia always deserves great attention, prompt diagnosis and treatment. Serum levels higher than 6 mMol/L are to be considered an emergency. There are three ways to oppose hyperkalemia:

(i) To antagonize cell excitability, a target that is attained by using calcium that works as a membrane stabilizer. Calcium is delivered intravenously either as calcium chloride or as calcium gluconate. Calcium chloride is three times more effective than calcium gluconate, but must be diluted to avoid thrombophlebitis. Both take some 15-30 minutes to be protective.

(ii) To drive potassium into the cells.
A way to do it is by infusing sodium bicarbonate to generate an alkalemia. A major limit of this approach is the sodium load that can be particularly risky in patients with ECF volume expansion, or defective control of sodium balance, e.g. patients with congestive cardiac failure or renal failure. A safer alternative is to infuse glucose and insulin in a ratio of 4 g/IU. Insulin activates a glucose/K^+ cotransporter and stimulates glycogen synthesis in liver and muscle cells. Therefore, insulin not only shifts potassium into the cells, but increases the so-called potassium capacity, that consists of the fixation of potassium to stored glycogen.

(iii) To eliminate potassium from the body using cationic resins loaded with calcium or sodium that are introduced in the bowel by mouth or by enema. The resins exchange calcium or sodium for potassium present in the intestinal fluid, 1 g of resin binding 1 mmol of potassium, and are evacuated in the stools. Their effect is slow but consistent because they actually reduce potassium content of the body. A very effective way to remove potassium is hemodialysis that is the obvious therapy of choice in patients on regular dialysis treatment as well as in patients with advanced chronic uremia and in patients with acute renal failure.

HYPOKALEMIA

The most common mechanism leading to hypokalemia is a sustained increase in distal sodium delivery. Diuretics are the main culprits because both thiazides and high-ceiling diuretics inhibit tubular sodium reabsorption in a site that is proximal to the tubular tract where sodium is exchanged for potassium. Indeed, diuretics resume all the mechanisms of hypokalemia because they deplete ECF volume and stimulate renin release and aldosterone secretion, and induce alkalemia (see Chapter 4). Alkalemia shifts potassium inside the cells and facilitates potassium excretion by increasing the concentration gradient between the principal cells and the tubular lumen.

Potassium loss is also caused by osmotic diuresis in diabetic patients with glycosuria and by disorders of tubular sodium transport that imitate diuretic treatment, i.e. the two hereditary syndromes: Bartter's syndrome (due to a defect of reabsorption of sodium, potassium and chloride at the Henle's loop. Symptoms are: hypokalemic alkalosis, high plasma renin activity, hypotension and resistance of blood vessels to angiotensin) and Gitelman's syndrome (hypokalemia, hypomagnesemia, hypokalemic metabolic alkalosis, hypocalciuria) that are the expression of a defect in furosemide-sensitive and thiazide-sensitive cotransporters, respectively.

Urinary loss of potassium occurs also in hyperaldosteronism, in particular in primary disease. Hypertension is a clue to diagnosis. Adrenal adenoma and adrenal hyperplasia are in general the most common causes of primary hyperaldosteronism, but there are rare familial forms, characterized by moderately high serum aldosterone levels that are lowered by glucocorticoid administration.

Gastroenteric fluid loss is a common cause of hypokalemia. Diarrheal fluid can contain up to 100 mEq/L of potassium. Less potassium is present in vomitus, but in addition to causing potassium loss, vomitus causes alkalemia and is associated with nausea that blocks food potassium intake.

Symptoms and treatment of hypokalemia

Heart disorders are the most frequent and risky effects of hypokalemia, that can cause cardiac arrhythmias and death. ECG changes are often early and isolated and consist of U-shaped ST tract depression and U wave presence, that can be misinterpreted as an ST prolongation when U wave is attached to T wave. Therapy has to be delivered when serum potassium is lower than 3.0 mEq/L. Moderate chronic hypokalemia, such as that caused by diuretics is treated by oral administration potassium aspartate or chloride. The latter is more effective but less tolerated because of its gastric side effects (burning pain, nausea). Potassium sparing diuretics and aldosterone inhibitors are often administered associated with thiazides. Food supplementation with potassium-rich oranges, nuts and bananas is advisable. Levels lower than 2.5 mEq/L are treated by IV administration, diluting potassium to concentration lower than 50 mEq/L to prevent vein irritation and phlebitis, and limiting infusion to rates lower than 20 mEq/h. In life-threatening conditions higher rates are indicated under serum level monitoring.

! TRICKY CASE? N. 2

A 70 year old patient with type 2 diabetes suffers from a severe urinary tract Infection for 3 days during which he scarcely introduces food and water and misses antidiabetic therapy. His relatives realize that he is drowsy and confused and bring him to hospital. Blood biochemistry shows very high glucose (5.6 g/dL) and hyponatremia (115 mEq/L). Serum potassium is low 2.1 mEq/L. Blood pressure is 95/65 mm Hg.
The trainee on call prescribes infusion of hypertonic saline (NaCl 200 mEq/L, 1 L in 6 hours), insulin, potassium chloride (20 mEq/h infused in NaCl 154 m/L), but in view of case complexity, he asks for the opinion of his tutor.
The tutor suggests a correction. Which of the following is the one the tutor should suggest?

ANSWER 1
Replace potassium chloride for potassium aspartate.

→

ANSWER 2
Replace hypertonic saline solution for one with lower NaCl concentration (130 mEq/L).

Disclosure:
In this patient coexist three electrolye/fluid disturbances, all caused by hyperglycemia. One is loss of sodium and water dragged to the urine by the osmotic load represented by filtered glucose escaping reabsorption. Another one is high plasma osmolality due to hyperglycemia, that shifts water from the intracellular to the extracellular compartment, the last one is hypokalemia due to urinary loss of potassium caused by increased distal exchange for sodium. ECF constituents, including sodium are diluted and low natremia in this case is not a valuable index of plasma osmolality. The complex scenario is an emergency that needs prompt interventions aimed to recover ECF loss, to reduce plasma osmolality and to normalize potassium. The first target is addressed by decreasing glycemia, i.e. by delivering insulin. As for ECF volume recovery, the infusion of a sodium chloride solution is correct but it must be hypotonic, otherwise it would further increase plasma osmolality. As plasma glucose decreases in response to insulin and plasma osmolality decreases, natremia recovers its role of osmolality indicator and can be used to decide the tonicity of saline infusion. Finally, administration of potassium as chloride salt at a rate of 20 mEq/h has to be done under control of kalemia in view of the complexity of its determinants (hemodilution, glucose cotransport driven by insulin, aldosterone levels).

CHAPTER 4

DISORDERS OF BODY FLUID PROTON CONCENTRATION

FOCUS ON pH

A sound tradition presents pH as one paradigm of how precise is the kidney in maintaining body fluid ion composition. In fact, physiological pH variations are of two decimal places and changes of one decimal place can have dramatic effects on vital functions. However, pH is not the direct measure of proton concentration but the "cosmetic" transformation of proton concentration (0.000000040 mol/L or 40 nmol/L) into its negative logarithm (7.4) a number much easier to handle, whose changes reflect exponential changes of proton concentration. Thus, a decrease of pH from 7.4 to 7.2 corresponds to a 40% increase of proton concentration. It is not a matter of wonder that such an impressive rise in acidity affects some biological functions!

METABOLIC ACIDOSIS

Metabolic acidosis is a pathogenic process that causes a decrease of plasma bicarbonate concentration. There are two different mechanisms that lead to a bicarbonate deficit. One is loss of bicarbonate from the body or a defect in tubular bicarbonate regeneration.

In these circumstances the balance between bicarbonate availability and its consumption is disrupted because bicarbonate is missing not because of excess acid load.

The alternative mechanism is an abnormal load of acid that exceeds the buffering capacity of the bicarbonate reserve. The acid load can be either generated by a metabolic disorder or introduced from outside.

The therapeutic approach is different in the two types of acidosis and for this reason it is mandatory to make a differential diagnosis.

HYPERCHLOREMIC ACIDOSIS

This form of acidosis is caused by a primary shortage of body bicarbonate reserve, not by excess acid load, and its distinctive feature consists of a rise in serum chloride concentration. Hence, it is defined "hyperchloremic". Serum chloride increases because chloride replaces bicarbonate as the anion that is associated with sodium reabsorption in the proximal tubule.

Renal causes of hyperchloremic acidosis

In chronic renal disease hyperchloremic acidosis occurs because the amount of filtered acid available for regeneration is reduced to a proportional extent with GFR. In most cases, a visible decrease in serum bicarbonate concentration occurs when GFR approaches 50% of its normal level, but this rule of thumb has many exceptions that depend on acid load and the extent of distal tubule defect. Primary defects of tubular handling of protons are not rare causes of hyperchloremic acidosis. They have been named from the tubular segment responsible for the defect, or ranked according to the time of their discovery.

Proximal tubular acidosis (type 2)

The disease results from a defect of bicarbonate reabsorption in the proximal tubule that lowers the level of serum bicarbonate at which apparent maximum bicarbonate transport is attained, from around 30 to 15 mEq/L. The pathogenesis of the defect includes genetic errors and acquired diseases. Fanconi's syndrome (see Chapter 14) is an example of genetic disease. Acquired forms are often due to drug toxicity, e.g. sodium valproate, or are caused by inflammatory or degenerative diseases that target the tubule such as myeloma. In patients that are not treated serum bicarbonate concentration is steadily 15 mEq/L, all filtered bicarbonate is reabsorbed, no bicarbonate is lost in urine and urine pH is acid as expected in a setting in which bicarbonate regeneration is intact and intercalated cells respond to acidemia. Oral supplementation of bicarbonate can correct blood pH, but causes loss of bicarbonate in urine and increases distal sodium delivery, two side effects that are responsible for major complications. Actually, the clinical picture includes symptoms that depend both on chronic acidemia and on its treatment. A consequence of chronic acidosis is calcium mobilization from bone that causes rickets in children and osteomalacia in adults. Furthermore, hypercalciuria can cause formation of stones and nephrocalcinosis. Bicarbonate treatment causes proximal bicarbonate escape and increases distal sodium delivery (bicarbonate here is always meant as sodium bicarbonate) that in turn raises sodium/potassium exchange and urinary loss of potassium. Potassium supplementation is necessary to prevent hypokalemia and its symptoms.

Distal tubular acidosis (type 1)

The first tubular acidosis to be discovered, this disorder consists of an impaired ability of the distal tubule to generate the proton gradient and hence to lower urinary pH. The disease can be an inherited defect of the proton pump or of the impermeability to protons of the intercalated cell wall. Multiple causes are acquired, including tubulointerstitial inflammatory diseases and amyloidosis.

A diagnostic feature is urinary pH higher than expected in a patient with low serum bicarbonate and acidemia. In this type of tubular acidosis serum potassium is low for reasons that are not clear, maybe because distal potassium excretion is facilitated by low intraluminal proton levels.

The symptoms of type 1 distal tubular acidosis are similar to those of type 2: in children osteomalacia and failure to thrive prevail, while in adults renal failure secondary to stone dependent urinary obstruction and infection.

Distal tubular acidosis (type 4)

In this disorder acidosis is part of a defect that extends to all the tubular cell functions that are regulated by aldosterone. In addition to the various disorders that decrease aldosterone release from adrenal glands, defective aldosterone activity can be due to inherited aldosterone receptor and signal transduction defects.

However, the most common cause of aldosterone block are drugs that inhibit the renin-angiotensin-aldosterone system such as ACE-inhibitors, angiotensin 2 receptor antagonists and spironolactone. The widespread use of these drugs is the reason why type 4 is the most frequent tubular acidosis in the general population.

Distinctive features of this acidosis are hyperkalemia and a preserved ability to produce low pH urine. Indeed the latter apparent paradox depends just on hyperkalemia, that inhibits ammonia production by proximal tubular cells. In the absence of ammonia, urinary acidity is not buffered and even low acid amount can reduce pH.

Hyperchloremic acidosis caused by bicarbonate wasting

Human bowel manipulates daily about 9 L of fluid, 6-7 of which are secreted, while the remaining are introduced by drinking and eating. With the exception of gastric juice all intestinal fluids contain bicarbonate in high concentration that peaks in pancreatic juice. Therefore, loss of intestinal fluid with diarrhea can rapidly cause bicarbonate wasting. Bicarbonate is present also in sweat, in concentration that rises with the rate of sweat secretion up to 20 mEq/L.

Therapy of hyperchloremic acidosis

Since shortage of body bicarbonate is the pathogenic mechanism of hyperchloremic acidosis, its treatment is straightforward: bicarbonate.

Bicarbonate can be given by mouth (1 g of sodium bicarbonate is 12 mmol) or IV. A basic rule of bicarbonate therapy is that it has to be started as soon as possible but it has to be continued slowly, with the aim of refilling the reserve in 1-3 days, depending of the amount of bicarbonate missing. The calculation of how much bicarbonate has to be given to normalize body pool assumes that bicarbonate has an apparent volume distribution that is (in liters) half of body weight (in kilograms). Then, assuming that normal serum bicarbonate concentration is 26 mmol/L and bicarbonate concentration in the sample is 20 mmol/l, here is the formula to calculate bicarbonate deficit:

$$\text{Bicarbonate deficit} = (Bic_n - Bic_p) \times BW/2$$

Where:

Bic_n is normal serum bicarbonate concentration in mmol/L.

Bic_p is patient serum bicarbonate concentration in mmol/L.

BW/2 is half body weight in kg.

Too fast bicarbonate infusion can cause significant side effects.

Bicarbonate is a sodium salt that expands ECF volume. The risk of sodium overloading has to be considered especially in a patient with renal or cardiac failure.

Plasma calcium is partly bound to proteins, partly free. At normal pH the two fractions are the same, that is 50% is bound, 50% is free. Increasing blood pH increases the fraction bound, reducing free calcium. Since free calcium is the fraction on which depends neuromuscular excitability, too rapid shifting of calcium from soluble to protein bound phase caused by fast bicarbonate administration can trigger tetanic jerks.

According to Bohr effect, the avidity of hemoglobin for oxygen depends on pH of the solution in which it is contained. Actually, in vitro a decrease in pH lessens the affinity of hemoglobin for oxygen and increases free oxygen availability. In blood, however, hemoglobin is contained in red blood cells that react to a decrease in pH by blocking the intracellular synthesis of phosphoglyceric acid. This reduction in acid production blunts the decreases in pH inside red blood cells. Thus, the cytoplasm of red blood cells is not as acid as ECF and too rapid bicarbonate infusion can switch intracellular pH to alkaline condition and cause a sudden fall of oxygen availability and symptoms of cerebral hypoxia.

NORMOCHLOREMIC METABOLIC ACIDOSIS

This form of acidosis is caused by an overload of acid that challenges the buffer capacity of the alkaline reserve. Bicarbonate is consumed, less bicarbonate is available as anion accompanying sodium reabsorbed in the proximal tubule and the quote of bicarbonate missing is replaced by the acid itself responsible for bicarbonate consumption. Tubular handling of chloride and chloride serum concentration do not change in contrast with what occurs in hyperchloremic acidosis.

Anion gap

Understanding the type of metabolic acidosis, i.e. whether the underlying mechanism is bicarbonate shortage or acid load, is necessary for a correct therapeutic approach. In principle serum chloride is the obvious diagnostic feature that differentiates the two forms, but the rough value of serum chloride concentration can be misleading because serum solute concentration depends on total volume of water present in the body, i.e. on body fluid osmolality. This bias can be avoided by pointing to demonstrate a newly added acid load, as it can be done by calculating the anion gap (AG):

$$\text{Anion gap} = (Na^+ + K^+) - (HCO_3^- - Cl^-)$$

Where: Na^+, K^+, HCO_3^-, Cl^- are serum concentrations in mmol/L. Calculation results in a normal apparent gap of around 18-20 mmol/L. In hyperchloremic acidosis the AG is not modified because the rise in chloride compensates for the decrease in bicarbonate. In normochloremic acidosis a "ghost" anion compensates for bicarbonate and the gap increases.

Note that AG obviates the confounding effect caused by changes in body water content because dilution/concentration involves to the same extent all ions.

Causes of normochloremic (high anion gap) acidosis

Their treatment

Lactic acidosis occurs in conditions of severe hypoxia, such as circulatory shock and low output cardiac failure. Oxygen shortage in muscles blocks mitochondrial pyruvate transformation into water and CO^2 and pyruvate is diverted to lactic acid generation by lactate dehydrogenase (LDH). Anaerobic metabolism of pyruvate can occur also because of excess muscle exercise, especially in people that are not trained. Toxic lactic acidosis can be caused by drugs such as phenformin in patients with renal failure.

Symptoms of lactic acidosis are those of acidemia with added muscle pain, cramps and fatigue, otherwise unexplained leukocytosis can occur.

Treatment must target the underlying cause. No benefit on major complications has been shown by bicarbonate administration.

Ketoacidosis is a life-threatening complication of type 1 diabetes that depends on inadequate insulin treatment. Energy production is shifted to lipid breakdown leading to ketone accumulation. Poor compliance to insulin prescription, acute infection and stress are common sparkling causes.

Symptoms include a typical fruity smell, vomiting, Kussmaul's breathing (hyperventilation with increased breathing rate and depth).

Diagnosis is straightforward in most cases and is supported by ketone blood levels higher than 3 mmol/L.

Therapy is aimed to lower ketone levels, but the dramatic condition demands taking care of fluid and electrolyte balance as well, because hypokalemia, hyponatremia and volume depletion are major death risks.

Diabetes team specialists should be involved in treatment whenever possible and bedside ketone and glucose meters should be available. Osmotic polyuria due to glycosuria causes impressive fluid loss, up to 10% of body weight, and the massive rise in distal delivery increases potassium sodium exchange leading to severe potassium depletion. Blood potassium levels underestimate potassium depletion because of potassium redistribution from intra- to extracellular volume caused by acidemia. Insulin is the core therapy. Bicarbonate administration is questionable because there is evidence that it raises further ketone production. The reader should consult specific guidelines to program the rate of infusion based on the patient's parameters.

METABOLIC ALKALOSIS

Metabolic alkalosis is a disorder that causes a rise in plasma bicarbonate concentration. It is the most common acid-base disorder but there is little awareness of its high incidence, in part because most cases are not severe.

PATHOGENIC ROLE OF ECF VOLUME DEPLETION

There are different causes of metabolic alkalosis, but all of them need to be associated with a common condition, that is ECF volume depletion, in the absence of which the rise in bicarbonate would be but a transient self limiting phenomenon. The reasons for dependence of metabolic alkalosis on ECF volume depletion are:

(i) Physiological bicarbonate reabsorption has an apparent maximum transport (Tm) that is attained at serum concentration just above the normal bicarbonate levels. Thus, trying to raise serum levels of bicarbonate by delivering a bicarbonate load is frustrated because maximum transport is soon reached and any further increase of serum bicarbonate is dissipated in urine. A frank alkalemia is not attainable by increasing bicarbonate in the body.

(ii) Bicarbonate reabsorption is driven by reabsorption of sodium in proximal tubule. ECF volume depletion increases proximal sodium reabsorption, consequently bicarbonate Tm is reached at serum concentration that represent a frank alkalosis.

CAUSES AND TREATMENT OF METABOLIC ALKALOSIS

The most common causes of metabolic alkalosis are vomiting and diuretics, followed by hypokalemia and mineralocorticoid excess.

The mechanism by which vomiting induces alkalosis is straightforward: direct loss of protons associated with negative fluid balance (vomitus + fasting), loss of discrete amount of potassium and moderate activation of the renin-angiotensin-aldosterone system.

Diuretics are a perfect "model"of "contraction" alkalosis. In fact, the engine of bicarbonate reabsorption in proximal tubule is a sodium/proton countertransport whose activity is increased by ECF volume depletion induced by diuretics. Furthermore, diuretics increase distal sodium delivery and aldosterone dependent exchange sodium/potassium. Last but not least diuretics activate the RAS system and aldosterone release.

IV infusion of isotonic NaCl solution quickly lowers serum bicarbonate by expanding ECF volume, decreasing Na bicarbonate reabsorption and causing bicarbonaturia. On programming ECF volume expansion one has to consider the effects of the maneuver on potassium because it will increase distal sodium delivery, sodium potassium exchange and potassium excretion.

! TRICKY CASE? N. 3

A 55 year old man presents fever, cough and dyspnea. His family doctor detects signs of pneumonia on physical examination and checks for leukocyte count and blood gas analysis. Neutrophils are 6,200/mm^3, P_{CO_2} is 27 mm Hg, P_{O_2} is 85 mm Hg, bicarbonate is 21 mEq/L, blood pH is 7.49.
Answer the following questions:

→

ANSWER 1
Assuming 26 mEq/L as normal serum bicarbonate concentration and body weight 70 kg. What is the bicarbonate deficit?

ANSWER 2
Which of the following therapies, if any, is correct?
a) Sodium bicarbonate powder 5 g at breakfast, lunch and dinner while eating over 3 days.
b) Sodium bicarbonate solution 160 mMol/L, one L by IV in 4 hours.
c) Doesn't need bicarbonate.
d) Ringer solution 500 mL by IV for 2 days.

Disclosure: The correct answer is c).
The decrease in serum bicarbonate is not a primary phenomenon, but the adaptive response of the kidney to respiratory alkalosis. Respiratory alkalosis and metabolic acidosis change CO_2 and bicarbonate similarly, but pH, as in this case, is illuminating.

TAKE HOME MESSAGE

1. The volume of extracellular fluid (ECF) is determined by the content of sodium in the body.
2. Do not misunderstand natremia for an indicator of sodium content. It is a concentration! In order to figure the difference between sodium content and sodium concentration, consider a 10 g cube of sugar and a watermelon. The cube is sweeter than the watermelon because it is 100% sugar, while in the watermelon sugar is about 7%. However, the content of sugar is higher in the watermelon because its weight is 5 kg, accounting for 300-350 g of sugar.
3. In most cases, peripheral edema is not a fluid retention occurring because the kidneys do not work. Rather, the kidneys work, but following deceptive instructions that are addressed to them by effective blood volume (EBV). Low EBV can depend on defective cardiac pump, redistribution of fluid from intravascular to interstitial space. In any case a mechanism that cannot be obviated by increasing ECF volume. Sodium retained has only the effect of increasing further edema.
4. Osmolality of a solution depends on the number of molecules of solute contained in unit solvent.
5. The kidneys regulate osmolality of body fluids by modulating the amount of solvent (water) not the amount of solute.
6. Therefore, disorders of body fluid osmolality are disorders of body water content.
7. Sodium and its accompanying anions represent over 90% of molecules present in extracellular fluid. Therefore, the plasma sodium concentration can be used as a surrogate indicator of osmolality.
8. In circumstances in which natremia is abnormal forget sodium to correct it. Think of water!
9. Disorders of serum potassium concentration are life-threatening.
10. On facing a potassium problem never forget to consider the interaction of potassium with pH.

11. Become familiar with changes in ECG induced by hyper-hypokalemia. They are often the first signal of potassium disorders.

12. Start treatment of emergency hyperkalemia with IV calcium salt to stabilize membrane potential.

13. Metabolic acidosis is a pathogenic process that decreases serum bicarbonate concentration.

14. There are two mechanisms of metabolic acidosis:

   (a) loss of bicarbonate or impaired renal regeneration of bicarbonate;

   (b) excess fix acid load.

   In type (a) bicarbonate lacking in serum is substituted for chloride (hyperchloremic acidosis). In type (b) acid excess itself compensates bicarbonate (normochloremic acidosis).

15. The two pathogenic mechanisms are differentiated by anion gap.

REFERENCES

1. J. Danziger and M.P. Hoenig: Role of the kidney in volume disorders: Core curriculum. *Am J Kidney Dis* 68:608-616, 2016
2. C. Wolf. Clinical Physiology of Acid-Base and Electrolyte Disorders. *New Eng J MeD* 392:1092, 1990
3. B.F. Palmer: Regulation of Potassium Homeostasis. *CJASN* 10:1050-1060, 2015
4. B.M. Koeppel: The kidney and acid-base regulation. *Adv Physiol Educ* 33:4, 2009
5. L.I.G. Worthley: *Osmolar disorders. Critical Care and Resuscitation*; 1:45-54, 1999

SECTION 2

GLOMERULAR DISEASES

CHAPTER 5

GLOMERULONEPHRITIDES

Glomerular diseases have been classified in several ways, according to histopathological criteria, pathogenesis, clinical presentation, but none is fully satisfactory because there is no straightforward and unique connection of histopathological, pathogenic and clinical features. Rather, they combine without following any general rule. Thus, we have decided to present in distinct sections the histological lesions, the pathogenic mechanisms and the clinical symptoms, then to describe how they combine and form nosographic entities.

HISTOPATHOLOGICAL LESIONS IN GLOMERULONEPHRITIS

The response of the glomerulus to inflammatory injury includes one or more of the following features:

- **Proliferation.** The term indicates an increased number of cells present in the glomerulus. Proliferation of mesangial cells and endothelial cells is named "endocapillary". Proliferation of the epithelial cells in named "extracapillary". Capsular epithelial cells grow in an asymmetric way forming a multilayered epithelial bulge that has inspired the name "crescent". Proliferation indicates local release of factors (cytokines, complement, coagulation products, immunoglobulins) that activate cells and stimulate their growth.

- **Mesangial expansion.** Mesangium is normally a pretty virtual space placed inside the capillary tuft that is directly in contact with the endothelial cells. In fact, the glomerular basement membrane (GBM) behaves as a continuous sheet that folds around the endothelium of the glomerular capillaries but after having covered almost the whole circumference bends to pass to a nearby capillary (**Figure 1**). This anatomical conformation permits that large molecules or molecular complexes skip the GBM barrier and pass into the mesangium, where they can evoke an inflammatory response. In particular, mesangial cells can grow and extend pseudopodes between the endothelium and the basement membrane of the glomerular capillary, an interposition that looks like a thickening of the basement membrane. The phenomenon is inappropriately named "proliferation" of the basement membrane. Sometimes interposing mesangial cytoplasm causes a splitting of GBM and a railway track appearance.
- **Glomerular capillary basement membrane thickening.** The phenomenon can be segmental and false because it is due to interposition of a mesangial cell as just described, or continuous when it is due to real growth of GBM around immune complexes deposits.
- **Spikes.** Spikes are GBM sprouts induced by subepithelial immune complexes (IC). Spikes grow around the IC, eventually incorporate them and fuse causing thickening of GBM.
- **Glomerular sclerosis.** A transformation of the delicate capillary tuft into the deadly uniformity of collagen. It can be segmental and focal. Segmental is a lesion that is not extended to the whole glomerulus, but is limited to segments of the tuft. Segment is a cluster of glomerular capillaries that is in contact with the same mesangial frame. Focal is a lesion that occurs in part of the glomerular population.

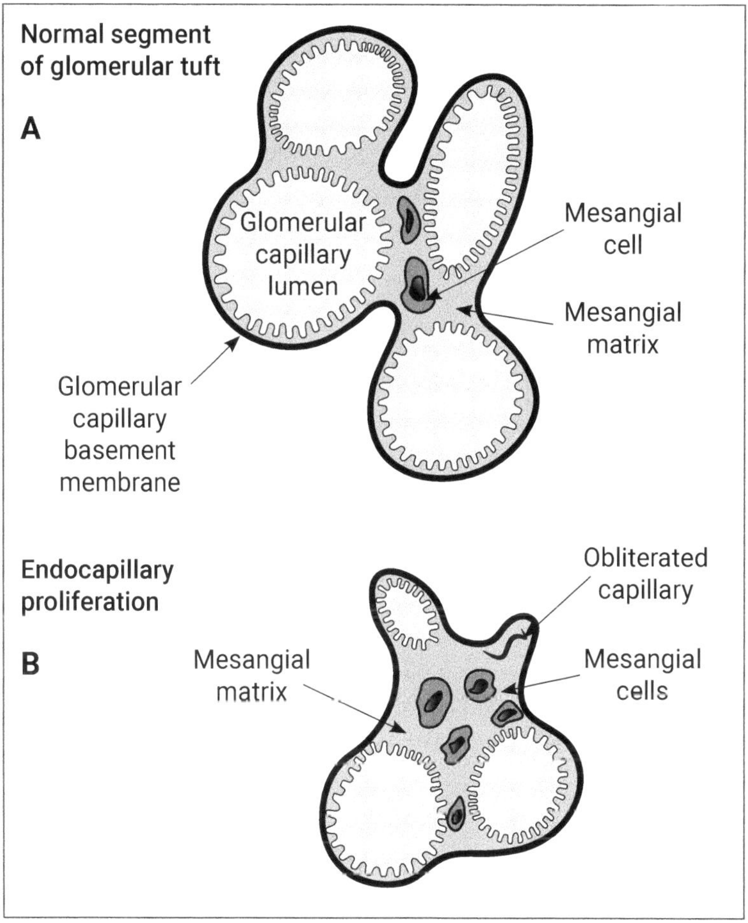

Figure 1 Drawing of a segment of glomerular tuft.
The central part of the segment is a narrow space similar to a stalk containing two cells and matrix (panel A). This space is the mesangium, from ancient Greek "meson" = "in the middle" and "angion" = "vessel". Mesangium is in direct contact with endothelium in a short tract of endothelial circumference that is not covered by the glomerular capillary basement membrane (the black ribbon that covers the outer side of endothelium). Circulating immune complexes (IC) can cross the endothelium and deposit in mesangium where mesangial cells, stimulated by IC proliferate, release cytokines and produce collagen. Progressive mesangial expansion obliterates glomerular capillaries causing glomerular sclerosis (panel B).

- **Podocyte bridging.** Podocytes that detach from the GBM and adhere with pseudopodes to the capsular epithelium. The phenomenon is a step to crescent formation.
- **Fibrinoid necrosis.** Death of capillaries or arterioles whose walls have the aspect of fibrin in tissue colored with Hematoxylin/Eosin (HE).
- **Exudation.** Infiltration of neutrophils.
- **Hyalinosis.** A particular form of arterial sclerosis occurring in small arteries and arterioles. The name comes from the ancient Greek word for glass and refers to the translucent homogeneous aspect of hyaline collagen that stains light pink with HE.
- **Mesangiolysis.** Lysis of the mesangial stalk causes fusion of glomerular capillaries resulting in microaneurysms associated with extracapillary proliferation. The picture is typical for the experimental glomerulonephritis raised by injection of anti-Thy1 antibody. In humans it is very rare, practically limited to HIV-infected people.
- **Nodular patterns.** Materials of diverse origin can deposit in glomeruli forming nodules that invade and disrupt the tuft. Silver stain helps in identifying collagen, e.g. nodules in diabetic nephropathy, while amyloid stains with Congo Red. In contrast, Silver does not stain light chain deposits.

ELECTRON MICROSCOPY AND IMMUNOFLUORESCENCE

Electron microscopy is not part of routine analysis of renal biopsy. However whenever possible a biopsy sample should be fixed with osmium tetroxide to permit electron microscopy if needed. Immunofluorescence is routinely carried out and adds invaluable information to histopathology, by detecting antibodies, immune complexes, complement fractions and coagulation products, and showing their site in the tuft.

PATHOGENESIS

IMMUNE MECHANISMS

- *Immune complexes*
  Glomerular inflammation can be secondary to deposition of immune complexes, that occurs with two different mechanisms. One consists of entrapment of circulating immune complexes, the other one of immune-complexes that form *in situ* (Latin, locally). In the latter case the antigen fixes to the GBM where it is later reached by antibodies. Circulating immune-complexes are much greater than antigens, thus they cross the endothelium, but not the basement membrane and localize in the mesangium or between the endothelium and GBM.
  Pathogenic antigens cross the GBM but are stopped by podocytes in subepithelial position where they are reached by antibodies. In situ IC can cluster forming "humps" and stimulate podocytes to add collagen to GBM.
- *Anti-GBM antibodies*
  This form of glomerulonephritis depends on direct attack to glomerular capillaries by anti-GBM antibodies. The antibodies cause capillary necrosis and release of growth factors that stimulate extracapillary proliferation and crescent formation.

UNKNOWN CIRCULATING FACTORS

In some cases of idiopathic nephrotic syndrome, proteinuria can be suppressed by apheresis, i.e. procedures designed to eliminate proteins from plasma. Based on this observation, it is reasonable to assume that proteinuria depends on circulating factor(s) that increase the permeability of the glomerular capillary wall. Indeed the nature and the pathogenic role itself of circulating factors is obscure because only a minority of patients with idiopathic nephrotic syndrome respond to apheresis and the same patient can become resistant in a relapse after having been previously successfully treated. Studies in children have given evidence for genetic defects that cause proteinuria with high penetration. These findings suggest that the variable presentation of idiopathic forms depends on the variable contribution of genetic and acquired factors.

CLINICAL PRESENTATION

Glomerular diseases can present with dramatic acute symptoms or be asymptomatic for a long time and be detected after the discovery of abnormal urine analysis, or loss of GFR, often as part of diagnostic investigations for anemia or hypertension. The possible clinical patterns are:

- **Nephritic syndrome.** Acute oliguria, macroscopic hematuria, hypertension, edema (facial). Diagnostic algorithm of its distinctive presenting symptom, i.e. hematuria, is shown in **Figure 2**.
- **Nephrotic syndrome.** Peripheral pitting edema, proteinuria >3 g/24 h, hypodysprotidemia (low albumin fraction, high alpha 2 fraction), hyperlipidemia). Diagnostic algorithm of proteinuria is shown in **Figure 3**.
- **Urinary abnormalities.** Proteinuria higher than normal (250 mg/24 h) but not as abundant as to generate nephrotic syndrome, microscopic hematuria, casts, leukocytes. Urinary casts are tiny cylinder-shaped particles made up of proteins, cells or cell fragments that have precipitated within a tubular lumen. Their detection in urinary sediment proves that their components come from renal tissue, for example they help in understanding whether blood found in urine depends on a renal disease or on a disease of urinary tract.
- **GFR reduction.** Active glomerular disease is often detected after the occasional finding of a rise in serum creatinine or urea. Anemia and hypertension are often present.

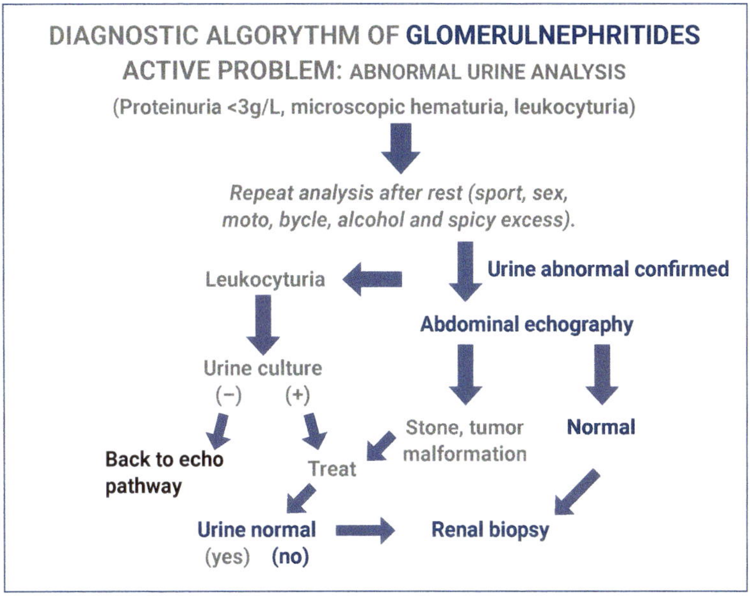

Figure 2 Diagnostic algorithm of urinary abnormities: *microscopic hematuria, low to moderate proteinuria and/or leukocyturia.*

The first step is to repeat the analysis and exclude non-renal causes: no active sport, especially sports with heavy contact (soccer, rugby, basketball...), no activity causing perineal or urethral trauma (cycling motorcycling, no sexual intercourse).

The second step is an abdominal ultrasound and in case of leukocyturia urine culture.

Third step: urine culture Is positive, trearad repersisting urinary abnormalities and absent urinary tract diseases lead to renal biopsy.

NOSOGRAPHY

POST-STREPTOCOCCAL GLOMERULONEPHRITIS

This disease is the paradigm of acute nephritic syndrome. Symptoms appear ten to fourteen days after an infection of *Streptococcus* beta hemolyticus group A has evoked an

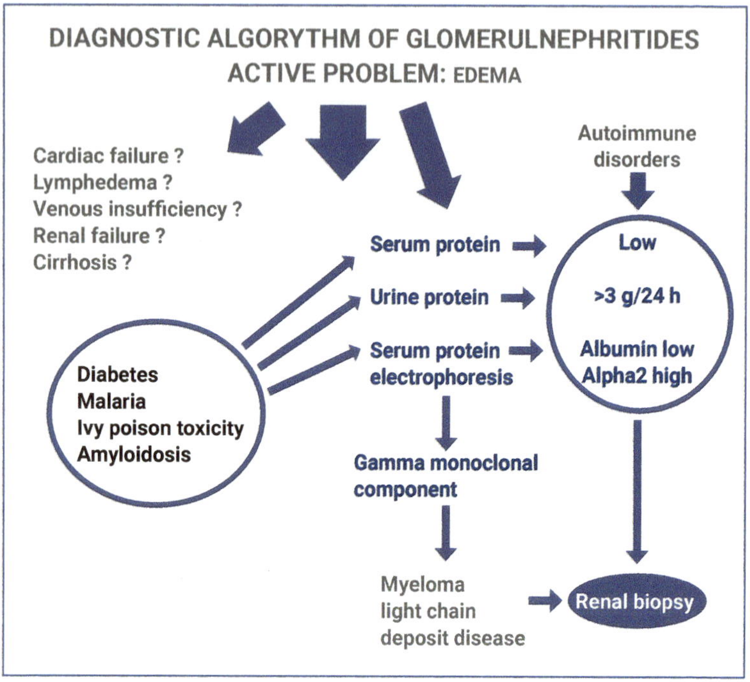

Figure 3 Diagnostic algorithm of peripheral edema.
First look for physical signs of cardiac failure, liver disease, venous peripheral insufficiency, lymphatic inflammation. Ask the patient for "foamy" urine (a signal of abundant proteinuria) and make a urine analysis. If you find abundant proteinuria, complete investigations for nephrotic syndrome.

antibody response against streptococcal antigen blocked in the subepithelial position. Gross immune complexes (named "humps") form in situ, activate complement and attract neutrophils into the glomerular tuft giving a picture of exudative inflammation. In most cases the disease heals spontaneously, but in its acute oliguric phase it can cause fluid retention, hypertension, pulmonary congestion and heart failure. These dramatic cardiopulmonary complications were noted in children with scarlet fever by R. Bright, a pathologist after which the disease was named.

MESANGIO- AND MEMBRANO-PROLIFERATIVE GLOMERULONEPHRITIS

A circulating immune complexes (IC) disease. In membrano-proliferative form mesangial cells extend pseudopodes between the endothelium and the GBM, creating apparent GBM thickening. Actually mebranoproliferative glomerulonephritis is a definition that encompasses disorders with distinct different features. The most common, type I, corresponds to the description just depicted, while type II presents deposits inside the GBM and a third variant has IC also in the subepithelial position. The most frequent clinical presentation consists of urinary abnormalities, i.e. moderate proteinuria, microscopic hematuria and casts. Many patients are asymptomatic and the renal disease is detected as part of investigations for hypertension or anemia. The disease progresses with variable speed to a final glomerular sclerosis. In a small number of cases glomerular capillary necrosis and extracapillary proliferation accelerate the loss of renal function.

A diagnostic clue of membranoproliferative nephritis is low complement level, but type I is associated with classical complement activation pathway while type II presents a persistent activation of the alternative one. A distinctive feature of type II is the presence of a serum immunoglobulin, named C3 nephritic factor, that stabilizes C3 convertase, accounting for persistent complement activation.

Most cases of membranoproliferative nephrits are idiopathic, but in a growing number of patients a secondary dependence on viral infections, particularly hepatitis C or neoplasms is found. Furthermore, this type of nephritis is often associated with systemic immune disorders, e.g. SLE.

Response to immunosuppressant therapy is poor.

Recurrence in renal transplantation is possible especially of type II.

IgA NEPHROPATHY

This is an immune complexes disease in which the antibody is an IgA immunoglobulin. The immune deposits are located in the mesangium, but sometimes they are found also in subepithelial position. IgA nephropathy is the most diffuse form of glomerulonephritis worldwide. A typical but not universal presentation of the disease consists of episodes of gross hematuria occurring in coincidence with an upper respiratory infection or a sore throat. These episodes remit spontaneously in a few days and are not correlated with progression of the disease. In the majority of patients the disease is slowly progressive and is diagnosed after detection of urinary abnormalities, e.g. moderate proteinuria or a rise in serum creatinine.

Membranous nephropathy

An in situ immune complexes disease often associated with solid tumors or infections that spread the pathogenic antigens. The subepithelial immune deposits induce growth of the GBM in the form of spikes that first bulge along the side of deposits then fuse over them resulting in an impressive thickening of the GBM. With time the removal of immune complexes can leave empty holes in the thickened GBM that look like it were moth eaten. The presentation is as nephrotic syndrome. The course is variable, from progression to renal failure to spontaneous recovery. The disease responds to immunosuppression in an encouraging number of patients.

The detection of membranous nephropathy makes it mandatory to explore whether it is associated with neoplasm or viral infection.

GOODPASTURE SYNDROME

Necrotizing glomerulitis caused by antibodies directed against the glomerular capillary basement membrane. Exactly, antibodies' target is alpha3NC1 domain of collagen IV. Renal biopsy shows extracapillary proliferation forming crescents that undergo rapid fibrotic transformation. Linear distribution of immunoglobulins along glomerular capillaries is found at immunofluorescence.

The antibodies cross react with the alveolar-capillary wall in the lung causing a necrotizing alveolitis that often dominates the clinical picture. The presentation includes gross hematuria, oliguria,

CURIOUS QUESTION

Urine discoloration

Urine reddish/brown discoloration can depend on hematuria, hemoglobinuria, myoglobinuria. Are you able to distinguish them having just a microscope and a centrifuge on your ward?

Answer:

Discoloration of urine caused by hematuria, often described as reddish, can present nuances that turn red to green fluorescent or dark brown, similar in appearance to Coca Cola. Indeed, color can be misleading to distinguish blood from free hemoglobin or myoglobin but uncertainty can be solved using simple means. By definition, hematuria is identified by red blood cells, that are detectable by dropping a film of urine on a glass and looking under a low power microscope. In the case of gross hematuria, red blood cells are visible without centrifuging urine. Hemoglobin can be distinguished from myoglobin by centrifuging blood to separate serum from blood and noting the serum color. In fact, both the molecules are released in blood from lysed red blood cells (hemoglobin) or muscle cells (myoglobin), but hemoglobin has a large molecule (64 Kd) and is partly bound to haptoglobin, so that it is poorly filtered and accumulates in serum, while myoglobin's smaller molecule (16 Kd) is eliminated from serum in a short time. Thus, in hemoglobinuria serum is dark and similar to urine while in myoglobinuria it is clear.

hypertension and a rapid loss of renal function (rapidly progressive glomerulonephritis).

Lung involvement can be life-threatening. Prompt aggressive immunosuppressant therapy can save at least part of the renal function. Apheresis can be of help.

MINIMAL CHANGE DISEASE

It is the prevalent cause of nephrotic syndrome in children but it can occur at any age. Its name reflects the absence of significant glomerular lesions at light microscopy and of immunoglobulins at immunofluorescence (see later). Electron microscopy shows fusion of the foot processes. In part of patients responding to apheresis a circulating factor has a pathogenic role. The disease responds to steroid therapy with complete remission of proteinuria in more than 90% of cases, but in a quite high number of patients it relapses in a variable time after steroid withdrawal. Some patients are steroid dependent, i.e. proteinuria relapses soon after the interruption of therapy. Cyclophosphamide, cyclosporine and rituximab are alternative therapies that can be used in cases unresponsive to steroid or presenting steroid dependence or severe steroid toxicity.

Hereditary forms of minimal change disease are described in Chapter 14.

FOCAL SEGMENTAL GLOMERULOSCLEROSIS

In its early phase this disease reproduces several features of minimal change disease: clinical presentation as nephrotic syndrome with no histological evidence of immune and inflammatory injury, some cases that respond to apheresis. Indeed, the two diseases could be the two sides of the same coin, one "good" and one "bad". Actually, in the very early phase of focal segmental glomerulosclerosis proteinuria can occur in the absence of any visible sclerosis in renal biopsy. However, the biopsy sample can miss sclerosis either because of its focal distribution or because the thin tissue section does not contain sclerotic segments. Sclerosis, initially confined within a few glomerular segments, expands progressively and in many cases eventually obliterates the whole tuft. Podocyte bridging, tuft adhesions to the capsule, extracapillary proliferation are bad prognostic indicators. Immunosuppression induces remission in less than half cases. Relapse is frequent and occurs also in grafted kidney.

CHAPTER 6

GLOMERULAR DISEASE IN SYSTEMIC DISORDERS

Glomeruli are often the target of injuries that involve the circulatory system, as expected from their extraordinarily high blood flow. The two kidneys weigh about 300 g (0.5% of body weight) and receive 25% of cardiac output, 90% of which flows through glomeruli exposing them to a possible huge load of inflammatory, immune, physical, metabolic and chemical insults. Furthermore, the peculiar structure and electric charge of glomerular capillary wall makes it a loose sieve that permits passage of big molecules to the mesangium but traps negative charges. Finally, native glomerular cells have peculiar phenotypes that can change when they are activated and transform into effectors of injury. Thus, mesangial cells can acquire macrophagic functions, podocytes and parietal cells behave as fibroblasts.

DIABETES

In developed Countries diabetes is the main cause of renal failure that demands renal replacement treatment. Indeed, such a high position depends on the dramatic increase of diabetes in the general population rather than on a high prevalence of renal failure in diabetic patients. Therefore, diabetes should not be assumed by default to be the cause of a coexisting renal disease. Actually, biopsy studies have shown that in 50% of diabetic patients with renal disease diabetes is not the cause of injury. Renal nephropathy progresses quite slowly, leading to renal failure ten to fifteen years after diabetes has been diagnosed. The very initial phase of diabetic renal disease is a functional change consisting of a rise in the glomerular filtration rate (hyperfiltration) that depends on a rise in filtration pressure. The next step is the phase of "microalbuminuria", a term that indicates a "small" (Greek = micron) excess of urinary albumin, ranging between 70 and 240 mcg/min. Microalbuminuria is associated with a thickening of the glomerular capillary membrane visible under electron microscopy. Finally, proteinuria announces the frank disease, in most cases associated with loss of filtration and hypertension. The typical histological finding of the advanced disease is nodular sclerosis, often associated with hyalinosis of glomerular arterioles. This glomerulosclerosis occurring in diabetic patients associated with proteinuria (up to the nephrotic syndrome), microematuria, hypertension evolving to renal failure is called Kimmestiel-Wilson syndrome. Primary prevention rests on strict control of blood glucose, while ACE inhibitors or angiotensin II receptor antagonists (sartanes) can slow the progression. Though in diabetes nodular glomerulosclerosis is the main culprit of renal failure, systolic hypertension, interstitial nephritis and atheromasia contribute injury and are possible therapeutic targets. In particular, hypertension has to be levelled down to less than 130 mm Hg.

SYSTEMIC AUTOIMMUNE DISEASES

Possibly all systemic autoimmune disorders can affect the kidney, with a largely variable prevalence and a wide span of severity. Glomeruli and arterioles are the main target of autoimmune assault but the tubulointerstitial system can be involved too.

arteries and of arterioles, tubular atrophy and interstitial fibrosis are additional findings that suggest that renal sclerosis results from tissue atrophy induced by chronic ischemia and hypoxia. An alternative mechanism of glomerular damage is glomerular hypertension, a physical insult to endothelium that would cause apoptosis and release of fibrogenic factors.

Renal disease caused by chronic hypertension has no specific clues that allow to state a sound etiologic relationship. Moderate proteinuria and microscopic hematuria are common and anticipate late symptoms caused by renal failure. Imaging, namely echography or plain abdomen Rx show a reduction of renal size and surface retractions due to scarring.

THE KIDNEY CAUSE OF HYPERTENSION

The kidney can cause hypertension either by releasing excess Renin or missing control of extracellular fluid volume. The former circumstance occurs in patients with renal artery stenosis, a pathogenic mechanism that has been demonstrated first by Goldblatt in an animal model. There are two different causes of renal artery stenosis, i.e. atherosclerosis and fibrodysplasia. Atherosclerotic stenosis is mostly due to an aortic plaque that has slipped over the opening of the renal artery. Fibrodysplasia consists of an abnormal growth of collagen fibers in the arterial wall. The phenomenon can occur in any part of the wall, intima, media or adventitia either in a single one or in various combinations. People involved are young adults, mainly female in which the hormonal contraceptive pill is a risk factor. Renal artery stenosis is the most frequent cause of secondary hypertension, potentially curable, in the general population. The diagnostic approach should be aggressive in young adults with sustained hypertension and include renal arteriography, not only because it is the best diagnostic tool but also because it can be followed by immediate treatment of the stenosis through stenting. In elderly people the disorder is suggested by an unexplained steep rise in BP or a recent resistance to antihypertensive therapy.

AMYLOIDOSIS

Amyloidosis is a disease caused by the deposition in tissue of amyloid, a protein that undergoes misfolding and polymerization in a way that gives rise to typical fibrils. Actually, the term "amyloid" does not define a single, specific protein but the fibrillar organization that can occur in several different proteins (presently over 50 have been identified). The altered proteins that form amyloid can be the expression of a genetic defect or be acquired. Here are described the two that are the most frequent culprits for renal disease.

One is formed by light chain fragments of immunoglobulin and is named AL. It occurs as a primary disease or in patients with myeloma or lymphoma

The kidney is affected in 50 to 80% of patients with AL amyloidosis, whose typical clinical presentation is nephrotic syndrome.

The second form is related with a chronic longstanding inflammation that causes the release of SSA protein (Serum Amyloid A). This form of amyloidosis is the most common worldwide.

Both AL and AA amyloidosis are systemic disorders that affect several organs. In AL, skin, gastrointestinal tract, heart, peripheral nerves are commonly involved, while AA rarely affects the heart and is associated with splenomegaly and the effects of hypersplenism.

The diagnosis of renal amyloidosis is straightforward by staining biopsy sections with Congo Red or detecting its birefringency under polarized light microscopy. Amyloid deposits are found in glomeruli and in the wall of arterial vessels. Amyloid has an amorphous aspect that may be misinterpreted as collagen in sections stained with EE, but in contrast with collagen it does not take the Silver stain. Often amyloid-loaded tissue sliced for microscope reading has a striped appearance, an artifact that suggests the diagnosis.

MYELOMA

Myeloma causes renal failure in about one third of cases. The most frequent mechanism of injury is the deposition of immunoglobulins in tubular lumen forming obstructive casts. Myeloma can cause renal failure also when it is associated with amyloidosis or release of light chains (K type) that deposit in basement membrane of glomerular capillaries.

LIGHT CHAIN DEPOSITION DISEASE (LCDD)

In this disease monotypic light chains deposit in subendothelial position and in mesangium forming nodules that are stained by PAS but not by silver nor Congo Red, a staining behavior that distinguishes them from nodules of diabetic nephropathy and amyloidosis. The disease is associated with myeloma and lymphoproliferative diseases, but in one third of cases is idiopathic. Monoclonal light chains are detectable in urine and serum with a 4:1 prevalence of K type. The dysruption of glomerular capillary wall causes abundant nonselective proteinuria and nephrotic syndrome.

! TRICKY CASE? N. 4

Loraine, an 18 year girl, suffers from frequent sore throat episodes with fever, muscle ache and local lymphadenopathy. As fever announces a new episode, she starts treatment with Aspirin 1 g and amoxicylline + clavulanic acid. 1 g three times daily. Symptoms last 3-5 days. The last episode occurred while Loraine was spending the weekend in Normandy, as guest of the grandmother of her best friend, Marie. Symptoms were as usual excepted for urine that was dark in two consecutive micturitions. Back at home in Paris, two days later Loraine talks the episode while sitting at dinner with her family. "Hey, it could be nephritis" says her sister Claire, a student of Medicine. Mom "Why didn't you tell us?" "Did you take your antibiotic?". "Did your face or legs become swollen?" asks Claire. The Dad "You said dark, but what was the urine color?" "Don't be so dramatic", Loraine answers to everyone, "Yes I took an antibiotic, one that was available in the house, rifampin. But I was well, no swelling, as for the color, it was reddish or more orange reddish".

→

Do you believe that Claire is right? Make a list of possible diagnoses and give them a priority.

Disclosure:

Dark urine can be caused by blood, hemoglobin, myoglobin, abundant urate excretion or drugs.

In this case the coincidence with a sore throat and fever suggests gross hematuria from IgA nephropathy. Other glomerular causes of hematuria such as post-streptococcal glomerulonephritis are excluded because there was no time lag between fever and dark urine. The urine color is an interesting point. Loraine was precise, defining it orange reddish, the very color given to urine by rifampin.

The two possible diagnoses have a similar probability share.

Let us wait for the next sore throat episode!

TAKE HOME MESSAGE

1. In most of glomerulonephritides glomerular inflammation is activated by antibodies localized in the glomerular tuft. Mostly, antibodies are components of immune complexes formed with non-renal antigens, but rarely antibodies are directed against an antigen of the glomerular basement membrane.
2. A distinctive feature of glomerular inflammation is the proliferation of glomerular cells.
3. A special pathogenic role is played by mesangial cells, cells with macrophage-like phenotype, that release cytokines and produce collagen.
4. Proliferation of parietal epithelial cells forming "crescents" (extracapillary proliferation) is an ominous prognostic signal.
5. Clinical presentation of glomerulonephritis is often silent, consisting of urine abnormalities detected by urine analysis.

REFERENCES

1. J. Floege: Primary glomerulonephritis: A review of important recent discoveries. *Kidney Res Clin Pract*; 32:103-110, 2013
2. S. Almaani, A.Meara and B.H. Rovin: Update on Lupus Nephritis. *CJASN*; 12:825-835, 2017

SECTION 3

RENAL FAILURE

CHAPTER 7

CHRONIC RENAL DISEASE

In this chapter we describe the pathophysiology and clinical presentation of chronic renal disease (CRD) that is not treated with renal replacement therapy (RRT), i.e. dialysis or transplantation. Actually replacement therapy generates specific problems that are not part of the natural course of renal disease. However, several aspects of uremic morbidity start before RRT but achieve particular relevance once RRT is delivered, so some content that is briefly anticipated here will be developed in Chapter 9 (dialysis) and Chapter 10 (transplantation).

DEFINITION

Chronic renal disease was staged about 20 years ago using glomerular filtration rate (GFR) as the only staging parameter. The resulting subdivision in 5 stages and the attribute of "disease" extended to subjects that had reduced GFR without any evidence for active injury to the kidney produced epidemiological evidence for astonishingly high prevalence of renal disease in the general population. Enthusiasm for what was announced as an epidemic of renal disease figured a new role of nephrologist as community specialist mainly involved in prevention. Further epidemiological studies showed that most patients with calculated GFR between 60 and 30 mL/min (stage 3) were elderly people or subjects with poor muscle mass in which GFR was steady and renal "disease" did not progress. It is now clear that a loss of GFR must be associated with signs of active injury to the kidney, such as proteinuria or decreasing GFR at follow-up to be considered the sign of a renal disease.

PATHOPHYSIOLOGY OF GLOMERULAR DYNAMICS IN CRD

Experimental studies later reproduced also in humans have shown that kidneys have a functional reserve, that can be elicited by delivering a high protein meal or infusing aminoacids. Protein and aminoacids provoke a rise in GFR that depends on afferent arteriole dilatation and consequent rise in glomerular plasma flow and glomerular capillary pressure. The phenomenon also occurs as the response to GFR decrease caused by chronic disease. Experimental studies have given evidence that the rise in glomerular capillary hydrostatic pressure associated with activation of renal functional reserve is actually a state of glomerular hypertension that causes glomerular sclerosis. Altogether, these observations provide novel support to low protein diet in chronic renal disease.

A distinctive feature of chronic renal disease is that in spite of GFR loss the kidneys maintain the balance between sodium intake and sodium output and similarly can eliminate normal loads of phosphate and urea. The phenomenon was described in the sixties of the past century by N.S. Bricker, who elaborated the concept that diseased kidneys behave as if their loss of function were due to complete deletion of a number of nephrons and the rest were intact. The "intact nephron" hypothesis offers a rational pathophysiological basis to the definition of chronic renal failure, as discussed in the next section.

CHRONIC RENAL FAILURE

An acceptable definition of organ failure is "a condition in which the organ is no longer able to perform its normal job". This definition fits well with heart failure, that limits normal physical activity and is graded according to patient's invalidity, but as applied to renal function it is not convincing. In fact, if we consider one of the pivotal tasks of the kidney, i.e. sodium handling, we find that patients with chronic renal disease that have lost 80% of GFR or even more are still able to excrete the amount of sodium contained in a normal diet and achieve the balance between sodium intake and sodium output. Renal sodium output is tailored to sodium intake by a feedback mechanism that perceives the changes in body sodium content and adapts sodium excretion through a complex system of effectors. The sensitivity of the system is determined by the extent of ECF volume change that is necessary to evoke the appropriate effectors. The human model of kidney, based on huge filtered volume that is almost completely reabsorbed is an extremely powerful and sensitive machinery that minimizes the change of ECF volume necessary to regain balance.

In fact, to dispose of the sodium load delivered by a normal diet, e.g. containing 5 g NaCl/day, it is sufficient that 3 out of 1,000 filtered sodium ions are eliminated in urine, and a change in dietary salt intake, e.g. from 5 to 10 NaCl g/day is promptly balanced letting pass to urine only 3 more sodium ions over 1,000 filtered.

Indeed, such a fine adjustment of tubular sodium reabsorption is achieved through minimal resetting of the effectors that regulate tubular sodium handling, and in turn such a minimal resetting is driven by a very low change of body sodium content, a change sufficient to operate feedback, but so fine as to be considered "physiological".

The feedback works also when a chronic disease reduces GFR. However, assuming that sodium intake is unchanged, the more GFR decreases the more fractional sodium excretion (FENa, the percent fraction of sodium filtered that is not reabsorbed and is excreted) must increase to achieve sodium balance. At some point in the progressive loss of GFR the FENa will rise disproportionately reflecting a strong inhibition of sodium reabsorption, and this inhibition will be made possible by a dramatic resetting of the feedback effectors, driven by an abnormal change in body sodium content. Epidemiological studies have shown that early on as GFR decreases FENa rises slowly remaining lower than 1.0% until GFR approaches 40-60 mL/min, then FENa rises steeply in exponential way. Based on these observations and on the consideration that FENa mirrors ECF volume expansion, it can be assumed that extracellular fluid volume (ECF volume) exceeds the normal limit when FENa starts peaking and that the correspondent GFR marks the border of renal failure, i.e. the point when the kidneys are no longer able to limit ECF volume changes within strict physiological boundaries.

While the loss of renal ability to maintain steady ECF volume gives some rational support to identify 40-60 mL/min as the GFR level that marks the border of chronic renal failure, it has to be acknowledged that the array of renal functions is so wide and diversified as to make it necessary to consider the state of renal insufficiency in relation with single renal activities. For example, calcium-phosphate metabolism starts to be abnormal at an early stage of GFR loss while water handling is generally sufficient at GFR levels very low. These diversities will be discussed in the respective sections of this chapter.

GFR MEASUREMENT

In classical physiology renal function, i.e. the rate of glomerular filtration, is determined by measuring the clearance of inulin, a substance that is freely filtered and neither reabsorbed nor secreted by tubule. In clinical practice inulin clearance is not feasible because inulin is exogenous and IV pump infusion is necessary to maintain steady blood levels while a catheter is placed in the bladder for timely collection of urine. Creatinine is a muscle product that behaves like inulin. Creatinine is a muscle product that behaves like inulin, i.e. it escapes tubular handling so that its clearance measurs GFR. The obvious advantage of being an endogenous product is in part obscured when GFR is lower than 15-20 mL/min. At low GFR levels, in fact, some tubular secretion raises creatinine clearance and overestimates GFR.

An additional shortcoming of creatinine clearance is the difficult and bothersome collection of urine for 24 hours. Actually today serum creatinine is used to calculate GFR, through formulas that give values normalized for age, sex and body weigth.

The formulas currently used are described in the **Box 1**.

BOX 1 Current formulas to calculate GFR (GFR_C)

Cockroft and Gault: this formula, proposed in 1976, was ahead of all the subsequent and is still popular for its simplicity. Its main bias is overestimation of low GFRs.

In males

GFR_c = [140-age (years)] x body weight (kg)/72 x serum creatinine (mg/dL)

In females the result is multiplied by 0.8.

MDRD: this is the acronym for modification of diet in renal disease. It reminds one of the original study in which the formula was conceived. Calculation is quite complicated but calculators are easily available online. The formula gives accurate results. Reproducibility, however, depends on the use of the "calibrated" method of creatinine measurement.

An alternative endogenous protein whose blood concentration depends on renal function is cystatin C. Cystatin C levels are not influenced by muscle mass and when available cystatin is more accurate and reproducible than serum creatinine.

Finally, clearance of radioactive tracers, e.g. Iothalamate or chromium allow precise measurement of GFR, but these methods are used predominantly in research settings.

CLINICAL PRESENTATION

Sodium retention is the obvious effect of GFR loss and causes a volume-dependent hypertension that in most cases is moderate and responsive to salt restriction or high ceiling diuretics. Although treating hypertension of chronic renal failure (CRF) by reducing excess ECF volume is straightforward, this initiative requires caution because volume depletion decreases GFR and increases blood urea concentration. The loss of GFR is functional and depends on reduced glomerular plasma flow in the setting of a dilatation of afferent arteriole that hampers glomerular autoregulation. Furosemide, the high ceiling diuretic most commonly used in patients with CRF, causes a rise in serum urea that exceeds the expected effect of hypovolemia, and depends on a direct effect on tubular urea handling that decreases urea clearance. Peripheral edema is not frequent in patients with GFR higher than 10 mL/min and when it is present it is often caused by heart failure or nephrotic syndrome. The reason for the late occurrence of edema is the self-limiting inhibition of tubular sodium reabsorption caused by ECF volume expansion.

Patients under renal replacement treatment, either dialysis or transplantation have a high prevalence of hypertension and are poorly responsive to treatment. In patients on dialysis the main cause of hypertension resistant to therapy is poor compliance to salt restriction associated with the intradialytic side effects of hypovolemia secondary to ultrafiltration, such as hypotension, muscle cramps and vomiting that limit the attainment of ideal dry weight (see Chapter 9).

Sodium depletion

While it is intuitive that renal failure causes sodium retention, it may seem intriguing that it can be associated with renal loss of sodium. Sodium depletion occurs in some chronic disorders that affect primarily tubular functions, in particular sodium reabsorption and are grouped under the definition of salt losing nephropathies. They include diseases that are very different as for ethiopathogenesis, e.g. tubular interstitial nephritis, cystic degeneration, genetic defects (see Chapter 13).

Independently of any primary defect in tubular sodium reabsorption, patients with chronic renal failure that have a high FENa and signs of ECF volume expansion can not reduce urinary sodium excretion to less than 30 mEq/L and undergo body sodium loss when eating a diet with very restricted sodium content.

Water metabolism/Plasma osmolality

In chronic renal failure, free water generated by the thick tract of ascending Henle's loop decreases approximately in parallel with GFR, but it remains sufficient to eliminate the load of water introduced by normal feeding until GFR falls below 10 mL/min. However, patients with GFR lower than 30 mL/min that abuse water are at risk for hyponatremia and the risk is particularly high in patients on regular dialysis treatment.

Similarly as for hyponatremia, also hypernatremia is a late complication in patients with CRF, at least as long as they are conscious, have free access to water and can drink, because thirst stimulates appropriate water intake. In contrast, patients that are in neurovegetative condition or that are nourished via percutaneous endoscopic gastrostomy (PEG) or central venous catheter (CVC) are at high risk because loss of water, especially from the skin, is easily underestimated.

Treatment of osmolality disorders in patients with CRF follows the same basic principle defined in Chapter 1, i.e. they have to be approached as disorders of water. A particular issue is the effect on free water clearance of high-dose furosemide used to treat edema in CRF patients with cardiac failure, cirrhosis or nephrotic syndrome. Actually, the item has been poorly investigated but there is some evidence that furosemide increases free water generation by raising sodium delivery to diluting segment, where reabsorption of sodium not associated with water is proportional to the sodium load that is presented.

Acidosis

In CRF acidosis results from reduced capacity of the kidney to regenerate bicarbonate, both because the amount of filtered buffers available for binding protons is reduced and as the consequence of atrophy and obliteration of distal tubules. Accumulation of anions, e.g. phosphate and sulphate increasing anion gap occurs when GFR falls below 20 mL/min and its contribution to acidosis becomes clinically relevant at very low GFR levels. Before dialysis treatment was available, acidosis often dominated the clinical picture and was a major cause of death in patients with terminal uremia. Treatment with bicarbonate must be delivered with caution to avoid side effects that include sodium overload, tetanic jerks and peripheral hypoxia (see Chapter 4). The principle is to start treatment as soon as possible and proceed slowly, not exceeding administration of 80-100 mmol of bicarbonate IV in 24 hours until the bicarbonate deficit is replenished (see Chapter 4). On handling acidosis it is particularly important to keep an eye on serum potassium, because acidosis shifts potassium out of intracellular compartment increasing the risk for severe hyperkalemia associated with potassium retention.

For acidosis in patients on dialysis treatment see Chapter 9.

Anemia

Anemia is common in patients with CRF and before recombinant erythropoietin was available it was a severe and invalidating problem. Not rarely, hemoglobin levels were 6.0 g/dL or lower, causing asthenia, breathlessness and cardiac failure. In addition to symptoms dependent on low blood hemoglobin, anemia was the indirect culprit for hepatitis B and C virus infection through repeated transfusions of blood in the absence of tests to detect viral contamination. The relevance of the phenomenon in the 1980s is demonstrated by Registry reports of the European Dialysis and Transplant Association showing a 30% prevalence of hepatitis C infection in dialysis patients.

The main cause of anemia in CRF is the reduced production of erythropoietin, a hormone that stimulates proliferation and accelerates maturation of bone marrow erythroid cells. The kidney is the principal source of erythropoietin, that is produced by fibroblasts allocated in the cortical interstice in contact with peritubular capillaries. Actually, in CRF erythropoietin blood levels are not different from those in normal people, but in the presence of anemia they should be higher by a hundred times.

Shortage of erythropoietin is not the unique cause of anemia in CRF. In the toxic uremic environment red blood cells are victims of a subtle hemolytic process that decreases their average life span. Furthermore, in patients on regular dialysis treatment some blood is lost in the extracorporeal circuit and the nutritional state is often deficient in vitamins. Bone marrow fibrosis caused by secondary hyperparathyroidism is a further cause of anemia.

Recombinant erythropoietin has dramatically changed the scenario of anemia in CRF patients, but its use is not free of side effects and its therapeutic target is not to normalize hemoglobin levels because they cause hypertension and increase the risk for thrombosis. Because of these side effects the target of treatment with erythropoietin is not to raise hemoglobin levels within the normal range, but to maintain them between 11 and 12 g/dL. Resistance to treatment in most cases depends on iron deficiency that can be missed in patients on dialysis in which bioincompatibility causes a chronic inflammation and accumulation of iron in ferritin overloaded macrophages (see Chapter 9).

Mineral and bone disorder

Chronic renal disease is associated with a multifactorial bone disorder that has been defined for decades "osteodystrophy", a name that appropriately distinguishes as a unique nosographic entity the combination of pathogenic mechanisms, histological changes and clinical aspects contributing renal bone disease. Some ten years ago, a referential group of experts proposed to change the definition "osteodystrophy" into "chronic renal disease – bone and mineral disorder" and to limit the former term to histopathology findings.

The bone disease that occurs in renal patients is the crossing point of several pathogenic roads that can be distinguished in.

(i) defective disposal of phosphate;
(ii) vitamin D shortage;
(iii) bioincompatibillity of dialysis;
(iv) drug side effects.

These pathogenic factors interact making the final result a melting pot with a variable content but always a peculiar taste.

Hyperparathyroidism

Phosphate is a waste product derived mainly from proteins. Its serum concentration is regulated by parathyroid hormone (PTH) that modifies its renal excretion. As the amount of phosphate filtered by the glomerulus decreases following the decrease of GFR, serum phosphate concentration rises and stimulates PTH secretion, that reduces phosphate reabsorption in the proximal tubule and blocks further increase in serum phosphate. Indeed, phosphate metabolism, as just described, is an oversimplification because phosphate serum level depends also on its intestinal absorption that is regulated by calcitriol. Furthermore, a new determinant of phosphate turnover has been identified as the complex represented by the bone-derived fibroblast growth factor 23 (FGF23) and its co-receptor Klotho. FGF23 is produced by osteocytes and osteoblasts under control of PTH and calcitriol and behaves as an hormone. The interaction between FGF23 and its receptor is peculiar because receptor activation requires the expression of the transmembrane protein Klotho. Actually, Klotho rather than FGF23 receptor is the determinant that selects tissues responding to FGF23. FGF23 regulates phosphate/calcium metabolism and bone turnover, by:

(i) decreasing phosphate reabsorption;
(ii) decreasing 1,25 dihydroxy-vitamin D synthesis;
(iii) accelerating its enzymatic inactivation.

PTH and FGF23 cause bone fibrocystic remodeling that can be typically observed in hand radiography as subcortical microcysts and detachment of small cortical fragments. Brown tumors similar to those found in primary forms can occur. A characteristic X-ray finding is the rugger jersey spine, i.e. an appearance analogous to the stripes of a rugby sweater resulting from alternate dense and lucent bands. In patients on hemodialysis long-lasting stimulation of parathyroid glands can induce tertiary hyperparathyroidism, i.e. disruption of feedback regulation of PTH secretion by phosphate and calcium serum levels.

Treatment of hyperparathyroidism aims to block the two causes of parathyroid gland stimulation, i.e. hypocalcemia and hyperphosphatemia. Indeed, the two targets are rational but they have been addressed in a way that has been poorly successful while creating a new form of bone disorder, adynamic bone disease (see later).

Vitamin D deficiency

The final step in vitamin D activation, i.e. the attachment of a hydroxyl radical in position 1 of the sterane ring to form calcitriol, is operated by proximal tubular cells so that tubular atrophy and interstitial fibrosis that are common features of CRF cause a shortage of calcitriol that is many fold more active than precursors. Vitamin D deficiency impairs intestinal absorption of calcium and phosphate and results in osteomalacia, i.e in impaired osteoid calcification and bone renewal. Symptoms are bone pain mostly in the spine and legs, bone deformity e.g. leg bowing, fractures and muscle weakness. In children the clinical picture is that of rickets. Oral calcium loading, mainly as calcium carbonate, was the treatment for vitamin D deficiency until synthetic calcitriol became available and was widely delivered to renal patients with the double purpose to restore bone formation and to abate parathyroid gland stimulation dependent on hypocalcemia. Enthusiasm for calcitriol peaked when evidence was found that a high-dose IV administration directly blocked PTH synthesis. Actually, calcitriol was effective in antagonizing hyperparathyroidism but it had disastrous side effects. Increased intestinal calcium and phosphate absorption raised their serum levels to saturation, with consequent precipitation of calcium phosphate in soft tissues, particularly in the arterial wall and lung. Arterial calcifications added further risk for cardiovascular events (see later). In a minority of patients these were the cause of calciphylaxis, a dramatic necrosis of subcutaneous tissue and skin due to obstructive deposition of calcium in peripheral capillaries. Furthermore, inhibition of PTH was excessive resulting in blocked bone turnover, a disorder that was named "adynamic bone disease". Currently, availability of vitamin D analogues that selectively inhibit PTH synthesis without raising serum calcium levels and of calcimimetic drugs that abate the sensitivity of calcium receptors of parathyroid glands facilitate control of hyperparathyroidism, but over one third of patients on regular dialysis treatment still do not achieve full normalization of mineral metabolism. The main reason is little compliance with diet and drug prescription that frustrates the possible advantage of new drugs, simply because they are not used. Increasing compliance is a difficult task that requires family involvement, psychologist help, dietician follow-up.

Uremic disorders

Severe uremia is associated with a group of symptoms whose cause and pathogenesis is yet poorly defined. We mean pericarditis, platelet dysfunction, peripheral neuropathy, immune deficiency, gastritis, sexual and reproduction failure. Today they rarely occur in pre-dialysis patients and are rather observed in patients that receive a dialysis dose too low to eliminate toxic waste products that are supposed to be responsible for the symptoms. Interesting studies carried out in the 1970s found in uremic plasma peptides with molecular weight (MW) of 15,000 to 20,000 kD. The molecular weight of these waste products was intermediate between urea and high MW serum proteins. Hence they were named "middle molecules" that seemed to be related with uremic toxicity. Unfortunately, the causal relation between middle molecules and uremic symptoms has never been proved and interest in the topic seems to be turned off.

Pericarditis, peripheral neuropathy and immune deficiency

Pericarditis is a late complication of uremia that occurs when dialysis treatment is delayed or dialysis dose is low. Variable amount of effusion, often hemorrhagic, collects in the pericardial cavity. A harsh friction rub is audible, that becomes fainter as the volume of pericardial fluid increases. Pain is common and stabbing, it is localized mainly on the left border of sternum and is exacerbated by deep inspiration due to extension of inflammation to the near pleura. The risk of tamponade requires strict surveillance, especially when pericardial effusion is present in the anterior pericardial cavity, a finding that indicates a fluid volume of at least 500 mL.

Peripheral neuropathy causes an excruciating pain in feet plants, known as "burning foot".

Uremia impairs cell immunity, a phenomenon that is associated with a prevalence of Th2 over Th1 lymphocytes and a resetting of cytokine network in which IL-4 and IL-12 prevail over IFN-gamma and IL-2. The immune response is weak, the risk for infection is increased, while vaccination has a high failure rate.

LOW PROTEIN DIET IN CRD

Urea retention is the biochemical hallmark of reduced renal function, to the point that the clinical condition of severe renal failure is named "uremia". Indeed, early investigators of renal disease believed that urea was toxic and plaid a relevant pathogenic role. Based on this opinion it was obvious that a low protein diet was considered a cornerstone in treatment of uremic patients. Diets delivered to renal patients contained 0.6 to 0.9 g of protein per kg body weight (BW) and privileged food whose proteins were rich in essential amino acids, e.g. meat, milk and eggs, while food like bread and pasta made with protein lightened flour were used as an energy source. Now it has become clear that urea is but a minor culprit in uremia, being responsible for relatively minor symptoms such as gastritis, floating, nausea and vomiting that appear at very high plasma levels. Therefore, the past strict restriction of protein intake has loosened and diets with extremely low protein content that in the past were often the cause of malnutrition are no longer prescribed. However, proteins contain phosphate and sulphate that are the main source of diet protons. In addition, experimental studies have shown that bolus protein loading in a condition of renal failure induces afferent arteriole dilatation and causes glomerular hypertension, that can accelerate the progression of renal failure. Therefore, limiting protein intake in renal patients, but to a moderate extent, is still advisable.

Note: lab evaluation of urea in plasma can be given as blood urea nitrogen (BUN) rather than whole urea molecule concentration. Since the two nitrogen atoms of urea weigh 28 vs. the whole molecule weight of 60, one has to check the lab method in order to avoid misunderstanding. BUN values are the equivalent of about twice higher urea values.

CHAPTER 8

ACUTE RENAL FAILURE/ACUTE KIDNEY INJURY

While the concept of acute renal failure may be intuitive, a strict definition is not as easy, because of the arbitrary quantification of the amount of renal function that has to be lost and of the time in which the loss occurs. Furthermore, renal function can fall because of changes in dynamics of glomerular ultrafiltration without any injury to the kidney tissue, a type of failure that should be better considered a "dysfunction".

The traditional nosography of acute renal failure is based on the "site" where the pathogenic mechanism is located, i.e. in the circulation (pre-renal), in the kidney (renal) or in the urinary tract (post-renal). The main advantage of this classification is that it guides through a valuable diagnostic pathway, based on a strict connection with pathogenesis, as discussed later.

In 2004 a group of experts proposed to change the name acute renal failure to acute kidney injury (AKI) and a new classification was presented that was focused on severity, based on risk, injury, failure, loss of renal function, end stage renal disease, criteria that composed the acronym RIFLE.

In 2011 the KDIGO (Kidney Disease: Improving Global Outcomes) Foundation developed clinical practice guidelines based on RIFLE criteria. This new classification has the merit of being a tool for collecting epidemiological data and predict the outcome and impact of therapies.

Currently, both the classifications are in use.

TRADITIONAL CLASSIFICATION

PRE-RENAL FAILURE

The term pre-renal means that the pathogenic mechanism is located "before" the kidney, where "before" refers to the cardiocirculatory system. This form of ARF is defined also "functional" because the circulatory disorder does not produce any injury to renal tissue, but rather it causes changes in physical determinants of ultrafiltration.

Causes of pre-renal failure

Fluid loss is the main cause of pre-renal failure. Vomiting, diarrhea, sweating, plasma leakage from skin burns, hemorrhage, use of diuretics, are common causes of depletion of ECF volume. The extent of fluid loss necessary to result in renal failure is largely variable because the pathogenic effector, i.e. hypovolemia as severe as to abate glomerular plasma flow and filtration pressure, depends also on fluid intake. Actually, the risk for negative fluid balance increases in any condition in which fluid intake is limited, e.g. in post-surgery and intensive care unit (ICU) patients or patients that lack consciousness due to neurological disease.

Low effective blood volume occurs in circumstances in which peripheral blood perfusion is decreased as if the body had lost fluid, but ECF volume is not depleted, rather it is expanded. In these conditions the kidney avidly reabsorbs sodium in an attempt to recover euvolemia, but the sodium retained rather than expanding circulating volume increases edema. In these conditions effective hypovolemia increases the risk of acute renal failure.

An example is the fall in cardiac output caused by an extensive infarction in a patient with chronic congestive heart disease.

In nephrotic syndrome aggressive diuretic therapy can precipitate pre-renal failure because the loss of intravascular volume is too quick to be refilled by fluid shifted from interstitial space.

Hepatorenal syndrome depicts a scenario characterized by a marked splanchnic vasodilatation while intrarenal resistances are increased, a combination that causes renal ischemia. The syndrome occurs in the advanced stage of liver diseases. As for the cause of splanchnic dilatation, it is assumed that it consists of local release of vasodilator(s) produced by bacteria or by endothelial cells. Nitric oxide is presently the most quoted candidate to play the role of culprit.

Dysregulation of dynamics of ultrafiltration

Strictly speaking this kind of acute renal failure is not "pre-renal" but we present it so here because it consists of a functional form. Dynamics of glomerular ultrafiltration has been defined by as yet unrivalled micropuncture studies dating back to the 1970s. Briefly, they showed that the relative impact of the three determinants of ultrafiltration, i.e. filtration pressure, glomerular plasma flow and ultrafiltration coefficient depends on the activity of the afferent and the efferent arterioles. Some drugs that target glomerular arterioles and change their diameter by increasing or decreasing the activity of the smooth muscle cells present in their wall impact the dynamics of ultrafiltration and can cause pre-renal failure.

The inhibitors of angiotensin converting enzyme block transformation of inactive angiotensin I into angiotensin II, a powerful vasoconstrictor whose receptors are expressed in efferent arteriole. In the special setting of a unique kidney with a stenotic artery or of both kidneys with stenotic arteries the stenosis causes overproduction of renin and consequently high levels of angiotensin I and II.

The latter selectively constricts the efferent arteriole and the increased resistance at glomerular outflow raises glomerular capillary hydrostatic pressure and compensates for the low inflow pressure, maintaining normal filtration pressure. Blocking AII causes a prompt decrease in glomerular hydrostatic pressure and in ultrafiltration.

Catecholamines are active on both glomerular arterioles, but the effects of epinephrine and norepinephrine on glomerular dynamics differ, depending on the combined action on glomerular arterioles and total peripheral resistance (TPR). Norepinephrine causes a powerful constriction of the afferent arteriole that decreases filtration pressure and blocks ultrafiltration in spite of a rise in blood pressure caused by the increase in TPR. Therefore, use of norepinephrine to sustain blood pressure has a high risk for causing renal ischemia and it should be limited to circumstances in which shock is a life-threatening condition. The systemic and local renal effects of epinephrine are dose-dependent and less predictable but in general they oppose and compensate each other, i.e. the rise in blood pressure and the resistance of afferent arteriole rise proportionally, leaving the filtration pressure unchanged.

Diagnosis of pre-renal acute renal failure

The principle that guides the diagnosis of pre-renal failure is its functional feature, i.e. its dependence on reduced renal perfusion secondary to hypovolemia, in the absence of inflammatory, necrotic, immune, thrombotic or any else injury to renal tissue.

It is expected that a functionally intact kidney responds to severe hypovolemia by limiting to its maximum extent any further loss of ECF volume. As discussed in Chapter 1, ECF volume is determined by the content of sodium in the body, so that in the circumstances of pre-renal failure the kidney preserves and refills ECF volume by maximizing sodium reabsorption. Hypovolemia also stimulates vasopressin release and increases water reabsorption. Thus, a simple urine analysis gives sound diagnostic clues, consisting in low sodium concentration and high osmolality. Oliguria, i.e. urine output lower than 500 mL/24 h due to marked water reabsorption is associated with urine osmolality of 500 mOsm/kg or more.

Clinical presentation

Clinical signs of ECF volume depletion (see Chapter 1) will be found in the case of fluid loss dependent hypovolemia, while signs of expansion, in particular peripheral edema are present in the case of low EBV. Serum creatinine and urea are increased and urine output is reduced. As for the minimum changes in these parameters to be considered diagnostic, they have been the object of personal decisions until the implementation of guidelines based on RIFLE criteria (see later section), that propose a rise in serum creatinine of 1.5 or a decrease of GFR >25% and urinary volume <0.5 m/Kg/h for 6 hours. Also these limits are arbitrary, but they have the merit of representing an acknowledged reference that obviates terminology confusion.

Disorders of acid-base regulation and potassium metabolism are frequent complications of pre-renal failure but in most cases they are generated by the clinical events that also cause renal failure, e.g. metabolic acidosis due to bicarbonate loss in patients with diarrhea, or hypokalemia in patients with diuretic-induced ECF volume depletion. Rarely the severity and duration of pre-renal failure cause typical high-risk complications of acute renal failure, i.e. metabolic acidosis and hyperkalemia.

Treatment

Treatment aims to restore renal blood flow by refilling body fluid according to the type of fluid lost or by correcting the underlying defect responsible for effective hypovolemia.

RENAL ACUTE RENAL FAILURE

This type of renal failure, defined also "organic", is the loss of renal function occurring in a short time (hours or days) due to injury to one or more components of renal tissue. Renal vessels including glomerular arterioles, glomeruli, tubules and Interstice can be involved, often in combination. The insult to the kidney can be organ specific or be part of a systemic disorder.

General clinical presentation

The many causes of renal ARF contribute a variety of distinctive symptoms that we will discuss later.

Some symptoms are common and represent the "backbone" of clinical presentation:

- **Oliguria/Isosthenuria.** Oliguria (urine output<400 mL/24 h) is an early symptom, often the first that is noted, almost always present in ischemic tubular necrosis (see later), not always present in other forms. The injury to renal tissue hampers the ability of the kidney to change urine osmolality, so that it approximates that of ultrafiltrate (around 300 mOsm/kg). Similarly urine specific gravity is around 1,010, but on evaluating it, one has to take care that urine does not contain high molecular weight molecules, e.g. proteins that raise specific gravity but not osmolality (urine protein of 10 g/L, possible in nephrotic syndrome or myeloma, raises specific gravity from 1,010 to 1,020).
- **ECF volume disorder.** Symptoms of ECF volume expansion (see Chapter 1) are frequent and often are the reason for starting dialysis. Lung congestion can be missed at physical examination because of fluid accumulation in the interstice rather than inside the alveoli.
- **Hyperkalemia** is a life-threatening condition that occurs very frequently, being contributed by reduced potassium filtered, reduced distal sodium/potassium exchange, metabolic acidosis and a variety of additional causes that depend on the underlaying disorder (hemolysis, rhabdomyolysis).

Causes of renal ARF: acute tubular necrosis (ATN)

Tubular necrosis is one of the commonest forms of acute renal failure and one of the renal diseases most investigated in experimental models. Renal failure is caused by the death of tubular cells, that can be extended to variable tubular segments. Indeed, necrosis is not the unique mechanism of cell death, that can occur by apoptosis and regulated necrosis, a mechanism intermediate between the two. ATN can be caused by two distinct insults, ischemia and toxicity.

An intriguing question and the object of many experimental studies is why tubular necrosis results in a fall of GFR. Animal studies have shown that tubular necrosis causes a "no-reflow phenomenon" i.e. a severe renal ischemia that persists after normal systemic circulation is recovered and a similar post-necrosis renal ischemia has been evidenced in man by ultrasound doppler and angiographic investigations. Therefore, it seems sound that GFR is low because the kidneys are ischemic. As for the mechanism(s) accounting for ischemia, there are two reasonable possibilities. One assumes that glomerular ischemia is due to disruption of the tubuloglomerular feedback, a process that stabilizes glomerular filtration rate and sodium excretion. In brief, the feedback uses the macula densa, a short tract of the distal tubule located between the two glomerular arterioles, as a sensor that responds to increased distal sodium chloride delivery by switching a cascade of effectors that ultimately constrict the afferent arteriole and increase its resistance. Consequently, the glomerular filtration rate is reset and excess sodium excretion is prevented. In ATN necrotic cells of the proximal tubules fail sodium reabsorption and the ensuing rise in distal sodium delivery evokes afferent arteriole constriction, but the fall in GFR is not self-limiting because it does not interrupt increased sodium delivery that depends on missed tubular reabsorption.

Possibly a second cause of afferent arteriole constriction is tubular obstruction by necrotic cells detached from the tubular basement membrane forming debris and casts. Experimental micropuncture studies[1] have investigated glomerular dynamics in

1 Renal Micropuncture is an experimental technique that permits to access and study single nephrons or part of single nephrons in vivo. Animals, mainly rodents, are anesthetized, one kidney is immobilized and superficial structures, e.g. glomerular capillaries, peritubular capillaries, proximal and distal tubules are punctured with pipettes of 3-6 micron tip diameter maneuvered by micromanipulators under stereoscopic microscopy. Hydrostatic pressures are recorded by special devices, samples of peritubular capillary blood and tubular fluid are collected and handled with micromanipulators. GFR of single nephrons, resistance of single

acute ureteral ligation and have shown that stopping urine flow evokes a dramatic rise of afferent arteriole resistance that lowers ultrafiltration pressure close to zero. A similar phenomenon may be caused by intrarenal obstruction at tubular level.

Causes

ATN can be caused by two distinct mechanisms, ischemia and toxicity. Especially in patients of intensive care units ATN is associated with sepsis, but it is not clear whether Infections have a direct pathogenic role or contribute to ATN by their effects on fluid balance and systemic hemodynamics. Recent studies have shown that in septic patients apoptosis is a type of tubular death and this finding has been interpreted as sign of direct pathogenic role of sepsis.

Usually, ischemic ATN is the evolution of pre-renal failure (see Chapter 8) and occurs when renal blood flow is too low to provide sufficient oxygen and nutrients to prevent cell death. Toxic ATN is caused by endogenous products such as myoglobin or by exogenous substances that form an ever growing list. The toxicity can be direct or the effect of a hypersensitivity reaction, i.e. tubulointerstitial nephritis. Medication, in particular antibiotics and antineoplastic drugs, Rx contrast media, non-steroidal anti-inflammatory agents are the major categories causing toxic ATN. The number of drugs and of biological or chemical substances that are reported to be nephrotoxic is constantly growing and are reported in accessible institutional data base. Here following we report spot information on some specific causes of toxic ATN.

- **Hemoglobinuria/Myoglobinuria.** Massive intravascular hemolysis is associated with hemoglobinuria and cast formation that can obstruct tubular lumen causing acute renal failure, but recently it

afferent and efferent arterioles, electrolyte concentration along single tubules are measured. Micropuncture has given an invaluable contribution to understanding most important aspects of renal function, from dynamics of ultrafiltration, to autoregulation, tubuloglomerular balance, sodium and potassium handling, water handling.

has been shown that hemoglobin has an additional pathogenic mechanism, i.e. that it drives oxidative reactions that cause tubular cell death. Myoglobinuria occurs after rhabdomyolysis, in acute alcohol toxicity or as a toxic effect of statins. Myoglobin precipitation is facilitated by low pH in distal tubule. Some toxic drugs cause typical changes, e.g. isometric vacuolization induced by cyclosporine. A common effect of hemoglobinuria and myoglobinuria is urine discoloration to a brown/red color. A simple way to distinguish whether hemoglobin or myoglobin is responsible is to check serum color. Hemoglobin accumulates in serum because its molecular mass (65 kDa) is too large to cross the glomerular barrier and only a small amount is eliminated in urine. In contrast, myoglobin (16.4 kDa) is filtered and rapidly cleared. Thus in hemoglobinuria but not in myoglobinuria serum is discolored.

- **Antibiotics.** Aminoglycoside toxicity is direct and proportional to drug load. Adapting the dose to body mass and renal function can prevent from renal damage. Beta-lactam antibiotics induce a tubulointerstitial nephritis as part of a hypersensitivity reaction that often causes also a maculo-papular eruption.

Histopathology

At a glance tubular dilatation and interstitial edema are noted. Several tubular cells have lost their nucleus and detached cells, cell fragments and debris are present in the lumen and form casts. Indeed, the extension of these findings is very variable, since they can be present in the great majority of the tubules without any distinctive localization or be localized in limited tubular tracts, in the distal part of tubule. Interstitial cell infiltration is common in tubulointerstitial nephritis and includes mononuclear cells, neutrophils and eosinophils. In the recovery phase one can find occasional mitotic cells.

Clinical course

Timely diagnosis of pre-renal failure permits recovery of effective blood volume and prevention of ischemic ATN. Once necrosis has occurred, renal failure persists for variable time, depending on age, nutritional condition, concurrent morbidity and the severity of injury. In most cases recovery starts 10-14 days after the diagnosis of ARF and is complete within one month. ATN is a severe disease associated with the death of over 50% of patients, a figure that has not changed for the last 20 years in spite of the progress of medicine. Actually, in most cases death is due to the disease that causes ATN rather than to ATN itself. However, ATN presents clinical features that are at high risk for death, e.g., hyperkalemia and fluid overload, two complications that occur especially in oliguric patients. In addition to retention, the shift of potassium out of the intracellular compartment due to acidosis and release of potassium caused by rhabdomyolysis or hemolysis, are risk factors for severe hyperkalemia (see Chapter 3). Volume expansion can raise blood pressure, while the blocking of erythropoietin synthesis causes anemia, two complications that impose a work overload on heart and can cause symptoms of cardiac failure. A clinical aspect often neglected is the catabolic state caused by ATN itself and/or by the underlaying disorder. In fact, nutrition deserves major attention as one important determinant of prognosis. Helping nutrition is a pivotal therapeutic duty, often the one that is lifesaving. While the symptoms just described have the highest prevalence, any dysfunction caused by renal failure can occur and have variable impact on patient's outcome. Thus, disorders of osmolality, immunodeficiency, acidosis are frequently present and sometimes they dominate clinical picture.

Acute renal failure caused by glomerular disease

Acute nephritic syndrome characterized by gross hematuria, oliguria, hypertension and edema (often facial) is the clinical presentation of ARF caused by glomerulonephritis.

Post-streptococcal nephritis was described first in London by Bright (hence its name Bright's disease) during an epidemics of scarlet fever. The disease spread in children with a very severe course and many children died with respiratory failure due to fluid overload. Presently, this form of renal disease is quite rare in developed countries and its course is mostly benign. In fact, only a minority of patients fit the definition of ARF. In contrast, poststreptococcal nephritis is the commonest cause of acute renal failure in developing countries, representing up to 50% of all cases. Streptococcal infection is usually in the form of a sore throat. Complement activation recruits neutrophils that infiltrate the glomerular tuft giving rise to an exudative glomerulonephritis.

Diagnosis is based on history, isolation of Streptococcus Beta Haemolyticus Group A from a pharyngeal swab, clinical presentation of nephritic syndrome and renal biopsy. Biopsy will show an intracapillary proliferation with prevalence of neutrophils, at immunofluorescence subepithelial deposits of immune complexes and complement.

The disease heals by itself, the "acute" symptoms disappear in two-three weeks, while microscopic hematuria and modest proteinuria can persist for years.

IgA nephropathy

This definition covers a variety of clinical presentations that share a common immunohistopathological feature i.e. glomerular deposits of IgA-containing immunocomplexes. The most frequent course is that of a slowly progressive disease and the corresponding histologic lesion is endocapillary proliferation, but rarely can it assume the aggressive behavior of rapidly progressive nephritis with extracapillary proliferation, crescent formation and glomerular capillary necrosis. In these patients gross hematuria is associated with oliguria, hypertension and a steep increase in serum creatinine, a dramatic scenario well distinguished from the recurrent episodes of hematuria evoked by upper respiratory infections that resolve in a few days.

Anti-glomerular basement membrane antibody nephritis

This is an immune disease in which the kidney is the direct target of antibodies that point to an antigen located in the glomerular capillary basement membrane. Antibodies cause a necrotizing glomerulitis, recruitment of mononuclear cells and neutrophils, activation of podocytes and epithelial parietal cells, release of cytokines and growth factors. The typical expression of this injury is the "crescent" formed by a mixed cell population that includes parietal epithelial cells and variable number of podocyte-derived cells and monocyte/macrophage cells. The crescent grows invading Bowman's space and undergoes a rapid loss of cells that are replaced by collagen. Similarly, the glomerular tuft pressed by crescent's growth and wasted by necrotic capillary disruption undergoes obliteration.

In most cases the disease occurs as the Goodpasture's syndrome that involves the lung in addition to the kidney. The renal antigen against which the pathogenic antibodies are directed, i.e. the alpha-3 chain of type IV collagen is expressed also in alveolar capillaries. Antibodies cause a necrotizing hemorrhagic alveolitis that often dominates the clinical picture causing dramatic hemoptysis and respiratory failure.

Renal vasculitides

The term vasculitis indicates an inflammatory disease of vessels. Actually, renal vasculitides are a heterogeneous group of diseases that share renal vessels as common target, but have different pathogenesis and variable clinical presentation. Renal vasculitides are often heralded by an acute, dramatic decrease of renal function. Immunosuppressant therapy can induce remission in as many as 80% of cases but the course is characteristically relapsing and renal failure is the final destiny in the majority of patients with renal involvement.

ANCA-associated vasculitides

ANCA-associated vasculitides are three distinct disorders formerly known as micropolyangiitis, Wegener's granulomatosis and Churg-Strauss disease. In 2012, a consensus conference decided to abandon the historical eponyms and changed the nomenclature: granulomatosis with polyangiitis replaced Wegener's granulomatosis and eosinophilic granulomatosis with polyangiitis replaced Churg-Strauss disease.

The common feature that characterizes these vasculitides are circulating anti-neutrophil cytoplasmic antibodies. The discovery that on immunofluorescence the antibodies could be distinguished by their distribution pattern as perinuclear (p-ANCA) or cytoplasmic diffuse and granular (c-ANCA) was followed by the identification of the epitopes, myeloperoxidase corresponding to p-ANCA and proteinase 3 corresponding to c-ANCA. Then it was observed that the epitopes were related with clinical presentation, i.e. in patients with granulomatous polyangitis (formerly Wegener's disease) prevailed anti-proteinase 3 antibodies while anti-myeloperoxidase were prevalent in micropolyangiitis

Clinical features

In general, ANCA-associated vasculitides start with a dramatic attack that is directed against the kidney or the kidney and other targets, assuming the feature of a systemic disease.

Microscopic polyangiitis

The kidney is the main target of this disease, but other organs are affected, e.g. lungs, skin, peripheral nerves. Fever, joint and muscle pain, asthenia are common systemic symptoms. Renal symptoms include hematuria, proteinuria, oliguria and rapid loss of renal function. In about 50% of cases proteinuria is abundant and generates a nephrotic syndrome. In urinary sediment red blood cells and casts are common findings. Renal biopsy shows a necrotizing glomerulonephris with extracapillary proliferation and crescent formation. Fibrinoid necrosis of glomerular arterioles and interstitial infiltration of inflammatory cells is present in 30% of cases.

Lung is the second frequent organ affected. The lesion is a necrotizing hemorrhagic alveolitis that causes cough, hemoptysis dyspnea. Chest radiography shows bilateral opacities with a typical ground glass appearance at computed tomography (CT).

Skin manifestations occur in 40% of patients and consist of a palpable purpura that is the visible expression of a leukocytoclastic vasculitis.

Neurological symptoms are mainly caused by peripheral nerve involvement in the form of mononeuritis multiplex, i.e. a painful ischemic neuropathy that affects single nerves in different times and combinations.

Granulomatosis with polyangiitis (Wegener's disease)

This vasculitis is associated with c-ANCA in over 80% of cases. Its clinical distinctive feature is the syndromic involvement of the kidney, upper airways (sinuses, nose, larynges, trachea) and lungs.

Furthermore, a histopathologic clue that differentiates this disease is the presence of granulomas, i.e. inflammatory lesions that form around necrotic vessels looking like microscopic nodules hosting large plurinucleated cells of epithelioid origin, epithelioid cells and monocyte/macrophage in a fibrotic matrix.

Necrotizing inflammation of upper airways causing pain, hemorrhage and nasal discharge, sometimes associated with ear chondritis addresses the diagnosis that is confirmed by biopsy, usually of the lung or the kidney. Renal and systemic symptoms are similar to those of microscopic polyangiitis.

Eosinophilic granulomatosis with polyangiitis (Churg-Strauss syndrome)

This vasculitis differs from the previous ones because vessel inflammation occurs at a late phase of the disease rather than being a bursting start. In fact, the disease presents three phases, the allergic phase, the phase of eosinophil leukocyte attack and last the vasculitis phase.

The first phase consists of atopic manifestations, e.g. rhinitis or asthma, the second of an inflammatory reaction of eosinophils that can bring their assault against any organ. Lung, gut, heart, skin, kidney are the organs that are more frequently involved (30-50% of cases). Eosinophilia occurs due to a rise in circulating eosinophils, an infiltration of eosinophils into the tissue and the organization of granulomas with a prevalent eosinophil cell population.

The kidney is targeted by the disease in the last stage in which a necrotizing glomerulonephritis with crescents is part of a systemic vasculitis.

Therapy of ANCA-associated vasculitides

In 2016, therapy of ANCA associated vasculitides has been revised by a task force composed of representatives of international scientific societies and of care professionals. The task force has produced recommendations, the most important of which are:

- **(i)** Treatment should be initiated as early as possible after diagnosis at the new onset of the disease and in case of organ or life-threatening condition it should be aggressive, i.e. consist of cyclophosphamide or basiliximab associated with a steroid. Plasma exchange can be appropriate for patients that do not respond and are in a life-threatening condition. Less severe cases should be treated with methotrexate or mycophenolate associated with steroid.
- **(ii)** After remission treatment with azathioprine or basiliximab should be delivered for at least one year.
- **(iii)** Severe relapse should be treated as new-onset disease.

NON-ANCA ASSOCIATED VASCULITIDES

Here we give a synthetic description of the most relevant autoimmune disorders that can target renal vessels, i.e. systemic lupus erythematosus (SLE), thrombotic microangiopathy, hemolytic uremic syndrome and Henoch-Schönlein purpura (HSP).

Systemic lupus erythematosus

In systemic lupus erythematosus (SLE) the prevalence of renal vasculitis has been reported to range between 10% and 30%. The most frequent form is associated with immune deposits detectable with immunofluorescence or at electron microscopy, located in the subendothelial space and less frequently in the media. The vessels affected are small arteries and arterioles. The deposits by themselves are not always pathogenic, i.e. they can be present in the absence of tissue injury, a condition that is defined "uncomplicated vascular deposits".

Thrombotic microangiopathy

Thrombotic microangiopathy (TM) is a syndrome caused by diverse pathogenic mechanisms that present the same clinical and pathological features. The syndrome includes thrombosis of small vessels (in the kidney glomerular arterioles and capillaries), hemolytic anemia marked by circulating schistocytes, increased LDH and low haptoglobin plasma levels. In SLE TM often occurs as part of antiphospholipid syndrome.

TM occurs also in thrombotic thrombocytopenic purpura, a disorder caused by a defect of a disintegrin and metalloprotease with thrombospondin-1 motifs [13th member of the family] (ADAMTS 13) the enzyme that splits the "ultralarge" multimeric von Willebrand factor into smaller fragments. Defective ADAMTS 13 does not cleave normally von Willebrand factor (VWf), producing large active fragments that facilitate platelet aggregation and thrombus generation. The defect of ADAMS 13 can be inherited or acquired. In the latter case it can be either an autoimmune disorder caused by autoantibodies, or the side effect of drugs, e.g. immunosuppressants like cyclosporin, tacrolimus and everolimus. A form of TM that is classified as a separate nosographic entity is the hemolytic uremic syndrome (HUS).

Hemolytic uremic syndrome. Typical and atypical form

This disorder consists of a thrombotic microangiopathy associated with hemolytic anemia and a dramatic rapid onset of renal failure.

The *typical form* occurs mainly in children affected by an enteral infection with particular strains of *Shigella* or *E. Coli* releasing a pathogenic toxin (verocytotoxin). Contaminated food shared with family members or children in a school community gives rise to an outbreak of gastrointestinal symptoms. HUS starts after 5-10 days of diarrhea usually bloody with abdominal pain and vomiting. Absence of fever is a diagnostic clue. Bleeding and capillary thrombosis in brain circulation give rise to neurological symptoms.

The *atypical form* is very rare. It has different causes, most of which are mutations in genes of the complement system, such as the gene encoding for Factor H that accounts for 30% of cases of atypical HUS. The genetic defect by itself does not induce disease, but it becomes pathogenic when its coded protein interacts with products of infective agents or dysfunctional factors of immunity and coagulation systems generated by a complex resetting, as it occurs during pregnancy. This disease occurs mainly in children, in which it represents the most prevalent vasculitis. Its onset usually follows an infection of the upper airways and is caused by the deposition of immune complexes in the capillary wall. The immune complexes are characteristically formed with IgA immunoglobulins that activate complement. Complement recruits neutrophils that invade the vessel wall, cause fibrinoid necrosis and die themselves leaving debris that characterize the vasculitis as leukocytoclastic (from Greek, it means "tending to destroy white cells"). The skin is always affected and shows a purpuric rash. Other common symptoms are arthralgia and bowel pain that can be associated with bloody diarrhea and an abdominal wall resistance to hand pressing, a symptom that is often misdiagnosed as peritonitis and causes emergency hospitalization. The kidney is affected in 50% of cases. IgA immune complexes deposit in mesangium and activate mesangial cells that proliferate. In severe forms mesangial proliferation is associated with necrotizing capillaritis, oliguria, macroscopic hematuria and a rise of serum creatinine, i.e. the clinical picture of acute renal failure. In these cases, renal injury can be irreversible and sometimes as severe as to require dialysis treatment. In general, however, patients heal.

Henoch-Schönlein purpura

This vasculitis is rare in adults, while it is the most frequent vasculitis in children. A purpuric rash consisting of palpable capillaritis spots and joint pain are distinctive features. The cause in unknown but the occurrence after acute upper respiratory tract infections and the deposition of IgA immunoglobulins in capillaries of tissue involved, especially in the kidneys and skin, suggest a derangement of immune response. Glomerulonephritis occurs in 40% of cases with a histopathological picture of endocapillary proliferation. Gastrointestinal symptoms occur in 40% to 70% of children. Abdominal pain can be severe and physical examination can mimic peritonitis and lead to emergency hospital admission.

The disease heals spontaneously but in a few cases recurrences take place.

Therapeutic hints

Specific recommendations for the treatment for lupus nephritis have been dictated by national and international societies of Rheumatology and Nephrology. Severe lupus vasculitis causing acute renal failure is invariably associatcd with a necrotizing glomerulitis, and its treatment is that recommended for the ongoing glomerular injury. Therapy aims to complete recovery of renal function.

A 3-day steroid bolus is followed by cyclophosphamide 1 g monthly for 6 months. Oral steroid associated with mycophenolate or azathioprine are maintenance therapies. Patients non-responders, intolerant or affected by serious side effects can be treated with basiliximab or calcineurin inhibitors.

No specific treatment for typical HUS, that is a therapy that blocks verucytotoxin, is available but complete recovery is possible if organ dysfunctions caused by vascular injury are promptly managed. Interventions can include dialysis, blood transfusion, parenteral nutrition and antibiotics.

In view of the variety of genetic defects that account for atypical HUS, research is faced with the need for developing therapies acting on single specific targets. The challenge is hard but some success has been attained.

POST-RENAL ACUTE RENAL FAILURE

Post-renal acute renal failure occurs when urinary flow is blocked by a sudden obstruction of the urinary tract.

Block of urinary flow can occur in many circumstances but in principle, the condition must be complete as it occurs for obstruction of a unique functioning kidney (solitary kidney) at any level of urinary tract or in the distal part of urinary tract common to both kidneys.

Solitary kidney is not a rare condition that can depend on congenital agenesis, surgical removal or ablating disease of contralateral one. A special condition is that of grafted kidney. Agenesis of one kidney has an estimated general prevalence of 3-4 cases/1,000 people, but this figure is possibly higher since the solitary kidney is often ignored until it is detected by chance following unrelated abdominal echography. It is not rare that on carrying out an echo exploration after the occurrence of a sudden anuria one finds an unsuspected bilateral ureteral obstruction. In such a case, it is obvious to argue that the obstruction occurred first in one kidney without causing anuria since the other kidney was still functioning and later in the other one (anuria did occur because the obstruction occurred in a condition of one functioning kidney).

The obstruction can really stop simultaneously urinary flow of both kidneys when it occurs at the urethral level.

Pathophysiology

While it is intuitive that blocking urinary flow will obstacle glomerular ultrafiltration, it may be unexpected that the mechanism is not a fall of ultrafiltration pressure caused by increased pressure in the urinary tract transmitted proximally through the tubule up to the Bowman's space.

In fact, experimental studies performed in a model of acute post renal failure, i.e. ureteral ligation, have shown that the response of the kidney to acute obstruction is not as simple as that occurring in a hosepipe when we stop watering our garden. Ligation of the ureter evokes a biphasic change in renal hemodynamics that starts with a striking dilatation of afferent arteriole. The ensuing fall in arteriole resistance causes a rise in glomerular blood flow and in glomerular capillary hydrostatic pressure. These adjustments contrast the rise of hydrostatic pressure that is transmitted backward from the ureteral lumen to the tubule up to Bowman's space and permit ultrafiltration to persist, even if at a lower rate than normal. The afferent arteriole dilatation occurs soon after ligation, but it lasts for a short time and after 24 hours we find a surprising inversion of vessel's response that consists of a strong contraction resulting in a marked increase of resistance. Glomerular blood flow precipitates to about one third of its normal value and hydrostatic pressure in glomerular capillaries is as low as to approach oncotic pressure. Such a resetting of the determinants of ultrafiltration makes the filtration rate hardly measurable and eventually results in a low hydrostatic pressure along all the urine collecting system, from the tubular lumen to the site of obstruction. Being aware of these pathophysiological events one is not surprised at not finding a urinary tract dilatation, i.e. hydronephrosis in the early phase of acute urinary obstruction.

Clinical presentation

Abdominal pain and abnormal urine are the symptoms that point to urinary obstruction as the cause of acute renal failure:

- Pain.
  - **(i)** Acute obstruction of the ureter, as typically caused by a stone, evokes a colicky pain that starts in the lumbar region and moves laterally around the flank, then descending to

the inguinal region and extending to the testis or the vulvar lip. Distinctive features of this pain are its severity and waiving intensity.

(ii) Prostatic obstruction can precipitate a urine retention that distends the bladder and causes a severe hypogastric pain enhanced by hand pressing.

(iii) Retroperitoneal tumors can cause a tearing ache but many are asymptomatic.

- Urine.
  Stones and tumors can cause gross hematuria. Anuria, i.e. the absolute absence of urine, is a distinctive sign of obstruction of a solitary kidney.

Diagnosis

Obstruction should be inquired as the possible cause of acute renal failure in any patient in which there is no clear alternative diagnosis. Imaging facilities, in particular echography, often make the diagnosis straightforward but it is not rare that a small stone in the ureter is missed and it is possible that the stone has moved from the pelvis into the ureter in the absence of pain. Furthermore, early after the complete block of urine flow the fall in glomerular ultrafiltration caused by afferent arteriole constriction saves the urinary tract from dilatation. Thus, do not discard obstruction as the cause of acute failure of a solitary kidney before having been assured by a CT scan and/or a retrograde pyelography.

ACUTE KIDNEY INJURY: A REVISED CLASSIFICATION OF ACUTE RENAL FAILURE

As already mentioned, the traditional classification remains a valuable instrument to help clinical practitioner in tracking the cause and the mechanism of the disorder. However, it cannot be used to determine risk factors and to identify predictors of outcome. The RIFLE criteria ranked the severity of the disease using as indicators the rise in serum creatinine and levels of oliguria. While this new classification proved useful in predicting outcome and understanding that outcome is determined also by subtle changes of the indicators, the arbitrary grading of the indicators and their susceptibility to factors not related with kidney injury has raised criticism and has led to a revised simpler classification (Acute Kidney Injury Network [AKIN] version).

The AKI classification has the merit to provide a method to collect epidemiological information, to stage the severity of injury and to elaborate indicators of outcome. As such the AKI classification is instrumental to epidemiological research and promises useful to program prevention and deliver therapeutic guidelines. However, to the purpose of the present handbook, the traditional classification remains a valuable tool that tracks diagnosis in a simple and rational way.

TAKE HOME MESSAGE

1. Chronic renal failure causes a multiorgan dysfunction involving cardiocirculatory system, bone, nervous system, gastrointestinal apparatus, coagulation and hemopoietic system.
2. As glomerular filtration declines the kidneys maintain sodium balance by decreasing tubular sodium reabsorption, that is, by increasing the fraction of filtered sodium that is excreted (FENa). Adjusting FENa the kidneys succeed in maintaining sodium balance until their function is as low as 10% of normal values.
3. Anemia, hypertension, acidemia, hyperphosphatemia, hypocalcemia, azotemia are common symptoms of chronic renal disease.
4. In acute renal failure urine analysis is a very important diagnostic support. Sometimes urine is discarded because "it was but a few drops". Instruct patient and personnel to collect and store it for examination.
5. Mortality in patients with acute renal failure is around 40%. Hyperkalemia and ECF volume overload are major risk factors for death.
6. Acute complete obstruction of urinary tract causes constriction of afferent arterioles and makes the kidney ischemic. Early after obstruction glomerular ultrafiltration is very low and the filtered fluid is reabsorbed almost completely. Therefore, no urinary tract dilatation is visible at ultrasound examination.

REFERENCES

1. T.K. Chen, D.H. Knicely, M.E. Grams: Chronic Kidney Disease Diagnosis and Management: A Review. *JAMA* 32:1294.1304, 2019
2. C. Ronco: Acute Kidney Injury, *The Lancet*, November 6, 2019

SECTION 4

RENAL REPLACEMENT TREATMENT

CHAPTER 9

DIALYSIS

Dialysis is a procedure that replaces the kidneys when their function is not sufficient to maintain life. From the invention of the first rudimentary artificial kidney by W. Kolff in 1944 dialysis has saved millions of uremic patients and today it continues to be the life-saving treatment for hundreds of thousand people.

The word dialysis derives from ancient Greek and means "separate by loosening". In chemistry it indicates a phenomenon observed in a bowl containing water divided in two parts by a semipermeable membrane.

When pure water is replaced by a mixture of crystalloids and colloids in one of the two parts, the membrane allows passage of crystalloids but not of colloids, thus crystalloids move across the membrane until their concentration is the same in the two parts. At equilibrium half of the crystalloid mass is separated from the colloids.

The process that shifts crystalloids along the concentration gradient across the semipermeable membrane is named "diffusion".

There are two types of dialysis, extracorporeal hemodialysis and peritoneal dialysis.

HEMODIALYSIS

OPERATING PRINCIPLES

The operating principle of hemodialysis is to circulate blood out of the body to a filter (dialyzer) where it flows inside capillaries whose wall is a semipermeable membrane. Outside of capillaries circulates a solution (dialysis fluid) whose composition is tailored to generate gradients that move solutes across the membrane. Solutes to be eliminated, such as urea, are not present in dialysis fluid and diffuse from blood to fluid, while solutes to be delivered to the patient, such as bicarbonate, diffuse from fluid to blood.

While diffusion is effective in removing solutes it is not suitable to correct volume abnormalities, i.e. excess ECF volume accumulated in the interdialytic period. Since ECF volume is determined by the amount of sodium present in the body, one could subtract sodium from the body using a dialysis fluid with low sodium concentration, but it would be an unhappy trade off exchanging volume control for risky hyponatremia.

Actually, ECF volume can be regulated using a pressure gradient to shift volume directly from blood to dialysis fluid compartment. The pressure gradient can be regulated subtly, being generated by the algebraic sum of a positive pressure in blood compartment and a negative one in dialysate compartment. This procedure is named "ultrafiltration".

While the operating principles, i.e. diffusion and ultrafiltration are theoretically straightforward, implementing hemodialysis in practice and making it more and more feasible has been a continuing challenge.

VASCULAR ACCESS

The first determinant of efficacy of hemodialysis is the quantity of blood (Qb) that circulates in the filter. The standard dialysis program consists of three sessions/week, four hours per session, with a Qb ranging between 300 and 500 mL/min, a rate that requires a powerful vascular access. In addition, vascular access must be permanent, safe and easy to be used, e.g. in emergency. The first device that conjugated an adequate Qb with a nominally long-term use was Scribner-Quinton shunt. It consisted of a flexible cannula connecting the radial artery with the cephalic vein. The cannula formed an external loop that could be split in two parts, one to be connected with the arterial arm of the extracorporeal circuit that brought blood to the filter, the other one returning blood to the vein.

The shunt worked quite well but with two major inconveniencies, infection and clotting. Furthermore, it limited use of the arm. Presently it has been abandoned almost completely and it is substituted for what is acknowledged as the access of choice, i.e. arteriovenous fistula (AVF). The standard AVF is created by connecting the radial artery with the cephalic vein so that the latter is perfused with arterial blood at high flow rate. In some weeks the vein adapts to the high-pressure flow, its wall thickens and its smooth muscle cell component grows undergoing “arterialization”. This change permits repeated puncturing and facilitates hemostasis at the site where two large needles are placed to draw blood to the extracorporeal circuit.

AVF has invaluable advantages over shunt and central venous catheters (CVC):

(i) the duration. It can work for years;
(ii) the length of vein available for positioning the needles;
(iii) the protection from infection and trauma offered by the skin.

Unfortunately, often it is not possible to create an AVF either because of arterial sclerosis or because the vein has been made unsuitable by repeated puncturing. Actually, patients with chronic renal disease should be recruited in an outpatient program, where expert personnel take care of sparing arm vessels in view of their future use as dialysis access. AVF created with good vessels can be used for years.

Also AVF is at risk of complications: thrombosis, aneurism dilatation, bleeding and rupture.

When distal vessels are not suitable to create an AVF, proximal vessels or artificial grafts bridging two distant vessels can be used.

Furthermore, two-port CVC specifically designed for hemodialysis are available. Catheter is mandatory in case of first emergency treatment, but also its use as access for regular dialysis treatment is increasing as prevalence in diabetic and elderly patients lacking suitable vessels is rising.

BIOCOMPATIBILITY

The "artificial kidney" was the first technical device that could substitute for an organ. However, it soon became evident that hemodialysis itself caused morbidity due to contact of blood with artificial bioincompatible material. In fact, extracorporeal circulation activates leukocytes and blood systems like coagulation and complement. Leukocyte activation occurs 10-15 minutes after the start of extracorporeal circulation and causes a transient leukopenia due to margination of neutrophils and monocytes in lungs. Furthermore, leukocyte activation causes the release of reactive oxygen species (ROS).

Also T-helper (TH) lymphocytes undergo a complex resetting of their subpopulations TH1 and TH2. TH1, i.e. the drivers of cell immunity are strongly suppressed, as shown by low serum levels of their nominal effector Interferon gamma, while IL4 a cytokine inhibiting immune response produced by TH2 is enhanced. This imbalance results in a blunted immune response that increases the risk of infection and decreases the response to vaccination.

Extracorporeal circulation also affects hemostasis and coagulation. Uremia is associated with a complex dysfunction of hemostasis and coagulation that on the one hand increases the risk of bleeding, on the other the incidence of thrombotic events. Hemodialysis adds complications because it needs heparin administration and causes contact activation of platelets, but at the same time it possibly removes toxins that are responsible for part of the dysfunction. As rule of thumb, in clinical practice dialysis patients should be personally tested for bleeding or clotting risk before undergoing procedures that challenge hemostasis/coagulation.

MORTALITY AND MORBIDITY ASSOCIATED WITH HEMODIALYSIS

This section is integrated in Chapter "Chronic renal disease" for items dealing with anemia, mineral metabolism and bone disorders, pericarditis, peripheral neuropathy.

Although hemodialysis is a life-saving treatment, life expectancy of dialysis patients is dramatically shortened. The main cause of death is cardiovascular disease, whose risk is twenty-five times higher in dialysis patients than in general population. There are many reasons for this phenomenon. One is the state of subtle chronic inflammation maintained by activation of leukocytes, coagulation and complement that causes release of effectors of injury to endothelium. In addition, atherosclerosis is accelerated by insulin resistance, hypertriglyceridemia and arterial hypertension. Furthermore, vascular damage is contributed by deposits of calcium phosphate caused by hyperphosphatemia. Additional culprits for atherogenesis are metabolic products that accumulate in uremic patients, e.g. L-methyl-arginine, and homocysteine. Indeed, causal relation of these products with clinical outcomes is not proved but it is suggested by association studies.

Amyloidosis

In patients undergoing regular dialysis treatment for many years a unique type of amyloidosis can occur, in which amyloid fibrils are formed by beta$_2$-microglobulin. Beta$_2$-microglobulin is expressed on the surface of all cells as part of the class I major histocompatibility complex. Contact with foreign material causes a steric change in its molecule and increases its shedding. Furthermore, cellulose derived membranes such as cuprophan, the least costly and most used worldwide, have a "cutoff" limit (the molecular weight that marks the limit of membrane's permeability) too low to clear beta$_2$-microglobulin. The combination of increased release and low disposal dramatically raises serum levels of beta$_2$-microglobulin and its modified steric conformation causes molecular aggregation in amyloid fibrils.

Beta$_2$-M amyloid deposits form in joints and bones, in which they are visible in plain X-ray as translucent areas. A particular clinical picture is the carpal tunnel syndrome, caused by amyloid deposits in the wrist channel that is occupied by the median nerve. Nerve compression causes paresthesia and burning, often excruciating pain in the first three fingers and the radial half of the fourth one.

Sexual dysfunction

In women in their fertile age menstrual irregularity is common and pregnancy is exceptional.

In men reduced libido and impotence are frequent. Erectile dysfunction has been reported in up to 80% of men on regular dialysis, an impressive figure that reflects its multifactorial pathogenesis. In fact, sexual dysfunction is contributed directly by vascular disease, neuropathy, drugs, diabetes, low testosterone levels, hyperprolactinemia and anemia, blood pressure instability, malnutrition and psychological inhibition.

EVOLUTION OF HEMODIALYSIS: HIGH FLUX MEMBRANES, HEMODIAFILTRATION, HEMOFILTRATION

For many years after its implementation as regular replacement treatment, hemodialysis was carried out with cellulosic dialyzers whose main advantages were low cost and easy assembling. Growing awareness of bioincompatibility of these membranes was a thrust to search for biocompatible materials. New synthetic membranes, i.e. polysulfone, polyethersulfone, ethylene vinyl alcohol, polyacrylonitrile, polymethylmethacrylate are now available that are claimed to be more biocompatible. Indeed, bioincompatible reactions also occur with these synthetic materials, but some studies have provided evidence that they improve patient survival. Actually, the effect of synthetic membranes on mortality can depend on improved dialysis performance, rather than on better biocompatibility. In fact, the main feature that differentiates synthetic materials is the possibility to create "high flux" dialyzers whose very high water permeability permits enhanced ultrafiltration rates and remove solutes by convection. Convection removes solutes by dragging them with water, so that solute clearance is proportional to the ultrafiltration rate. In turn, ultrafiltration is determined by pressure gradient and is independent of solute size and concentration gradient, so that convection is advantageous in comparison with diffusion in removing middle-high molecular weight molecules. Depuration of high weight molecules has been further potentiated by producing synthetic membranes with large pores that increase sieving coefficient.

Sieving coefficient of a given membrane for a given solute is the ratio between solute concentration in the compartment of ultrafiltrate and solute concentration in blood. It measures the permeability of a membrane to solutes and ranges from one (solutes with low molecular weight that cross freely the membrane) to zero (big molecule that is too large to cross the dialysis membrane).

Variety of high flux treatments

Clearly, high ultrafiltration rates would be rapidly self-limiting, being opposed by hemoconcentration, if ultrafiltered volume were not replaced by fluid infusion. The solution infused has a protein-cleared serum-like composition and can be delivered soon before blood enters (pre-dilution) or soon after it leaves (post-dilution) the filter. Both methods have advantages and shortcomings. Pre-dilution needs larger volumes of infusion fluid, it is more expensive and if associated with dialysis (hemodiafltration), it reduces diffusive clearance of small molecules because of its effect on concentration gradient. On the other hand it has less effect on hemodynamic stability and it prevents formation of so-called "protein cake", a deposition of proteins in membrane pores that decreases ultrafiltration and lowers the sieving coefficient.

High-flux dialyzers are used in various modes, e.g. combining convection with diffusion (hemodiafiltration) or just as ultrafilters without running dialysis fluid (hemofiltration). Furthermore, treatment can be intermittent or continuous and extracorporeal blood flow can be high as in hemodialysis or low and derived from a central vein (continuous vein-venous hemofiltration).

Generally, hemodiafiltration is delivered as regular replacement treatment intermittent as hemodialysis, while hemofiltration is used in critical care patients with acute renal failure.

Advantages of high-flux dialyzers

Utility of high-flux dialyzers and convective depuration are supported by a rational base but as yet not by a sound, strong scientific demonstration. As a matter of fact, patients shifted to hemodiafiltration from standard hemodialysis "feel better", a subjective statement that can simply express the better hemodynamic stability offered by the fine tuning of fluid removal made possible by adding infusion control to ultrafiltration. Furthermore, high flux convective treatment removes middle/high weight molecules and can prevent uremic complications, i.e $beta_2$-microglobulin amyloidosis. Similarly, hemodiafiltration would depurate so-called "middle molecules" that are thought to account for uremic complications such as pericarditis and peripheral neuropathy.

HINTS ON PRACTICAL MANAGEMENT OF HEMODIALYSIS

Control of body fluid volume

In most dialyzed patients ECF volume undergoes expansion in the interdialytic time. In the short term the gain in body fluid is measurable from the change in body weight so that accurate recording of body at the end of dialysis session and soon before starting the next one is all that is necessary to program the volume of fluid that has to be eliminated to recover fluid balance. The target of ultrafiltration is to reach so-called "dry weight", i.e. a weight corresponding to a moderate hydropenia. In fact, moderate ECF volume depletion rather than normal ECF is preferable in view of the fluid retention occurring in the interdialytic period. Determination of dry weight is pragmatic. The method consists of progressively reducing body weight modulating ultrafiltration until symptoms of volume depletion appear (cramps, hypotension, nausea, vomiting, abdominal pain, fainting) . Dry weight is assumed to be the lowest recorded before symptoms occur. Dry weight should be tested periodically because dry body mass can change in a time of months or even weeks depending on nutrition.

Hypertension is volume dependent in most of dialysis patients, but even if in theory it is curable by reducing ECF volume, in practice hypertension is adequately controlled in about one third of dialysis patients. The main reason for such a failure is that ultrafiltration empties the intravascular compartment at a rate faster than its refilling by fluid shifted from interstitial space.

The ensuing symptoms of volume depletion limit further removal of fluid from circulation and hamper attainment of dry weight. The problem is particularly present in elderly people and diabetic patients that frequently suffer from autonomic nervous insufficiency. Endowment of last generation dialysis machines with devices that track computerized ultrafiltration curves and operate feedback control of hemodynamic stability are of great help in handling the problem.

Hitching

In dialysis patients hitching is a common symptom that can be tearing, as witnessed by impressive scratching lesions. The main cause of hitching is deposition in the skin of calcium phosphate occurring in patients with high blood levels of phosphate. Risk of precipitation of calcium phosphate in soft tissues is increased by treatment with calcitriol, that raises intestinal absorption of calcium and phosphate. In addition to skin, arterial wall, lung interstice and eye can be involved. In some patients hitching is not associated with disorders of mineral metabolism. Hypersensitivity to materials of extracorporeal circuit, in particular to chemical products used to boost plastification is a possible cause, but often the reason is obscure.

Anemia

As already discussed, reduced erythropoietin (EPO) synthesis is the main cause of anemia in dialysis patients, but not unique, so that iron and vitamin shortage or bleeding are to be considered especially when a decrease in hemoglobin is not responsive to EPO.

Adequacy of dialysis

Adequacy of dialytic "dose" is first of all based on clinical evaluation encompassing the various possible morbidities associated with uremia and dialysis itself. Dialysis dose can be quantified using as index fractional clearance of urea. The index formula is:

$$Kt/V$$

where K is urea clearance of dialyzer, t is time of treatment and V is the volume of distribution of urea in the body, generally assumed to be 60% of body weight (in liters). The validity of Kt/V has been questioned. In fact the same value corresponds to diverse extents of depuration in people with different body mass (in patients with low body mass Kt/V overestimates depuration). In addition, it measures diffusive but not convective clearance and uses urea as the index product in spite of its lack of toxicity. Furthermore, it does not consider that different substances have diverse rates of vascular refilling from extravascular fluid compartments. In spite of these shortcomings Kt/V is a useful complement to clinical evaluation and is currently used as an advisable instrument to detect patients that receive an inadequate dialysis dose, i.e. those whose Kt/V is lower than 1.2.

PERITONEAL DIALYSIS

Peritoneal dialysis (PD) uses the peritoneum as a semipermeable membrane that separates blood compartment represented by peritoneal capillary network from dialysis fluid introduced in the abdominal cavity through a catheter.

Initially, in the 1960s to the early 1970s, before hemodialysis facilities were available for all incident uremic patients, PD was delivered as a rescue, second-class therapy. The procedure was rudimentary: a catheter mounted on a sharp-pointed metal rod was pushed into the peritoneal cavity through a small cutaneous incision, then fixed to the skin with one-two surgical points. One/two liter bags containing dialysis solution were connected to the catheter by a luer lock and were emptied into the abdomen. Fluid was left inside for 30-60 minutes, then it was recovered in the bag by gravity. Exchanges were repeated as long as possible and generally they were interrupted because of catheter occlusion. The patient was discharged from the hospital and was admitted again to repeat the procedure when severe symptoms reappeared. Such a rough form of peritoneal dialysis was going to be abandoned, as availability of hemodialysis and success of renal transplantation were growing, when in 1971 the simple but genial initiative of placing an indwelling catheter in the peritoneal cavity permitted delivery of a continuous treatment that could be performed at home by the patient or by a family member.

CONTINUOUS AMBULATORY PERITONEAL DIALYSIS

As just anticipated, the indwelling peritoneal catheter makes it feasible for a peritoneal dialysis continuous and ambulatory (CAPD) in which "continuous" means that dialysis fluid is present in abdomen uninterruptedly and "ambulatory" means that the procedure is managed in an outpatient setting at home, with active participation of patients and their family members that are trained for that purpose. In practice, dialysis fluid is introduced into the peritoneum from bags specifically designed for connecting with the indwelling catheter and it is left inside for a time variable from 4 to 6 hours, then it is discharged by gravity in collection bags. The cycle is repeated without interruptions and the number of cycles varies from 4 to 6/day depending on patient body mass and metabolic waste production.

Of course, CAPD can not regulate ECF volume using ultrafiltration. Actually, in CAPD excess ECF volume is removed by introducing hypertonic dialysis solution that drains fluid along an osmotic gradient. Hypertonicity is obtained by adding glucose (1.36%, 3.86% or icodextrine 7.5%).

AUTOMATED PERITONEAL DIALYSIS

A further step in improving peritoneal dialysis feasibility and efficacy has been the implementation of machines that run dialysis cycles automatically according to a personalized program. Automated peritoneal dialysis (APD) can be delivered in the night to the sleeping patient, an advantage that is particularly appreciated by people engaged in work.

ADVANTAGES AND LIMITS OF PERITONEAL DIALYSIS

The main advantage of CAPD and APD is that they are managed at home and avoid the boring and time-wasting access to a hemodialysis center. Actually, the first CAPD program was implemented in Canada to obviate transport of native Eskimo patients to a very distant Dialysis Center. An additional advantage is that devices necessary for carrying out PD, including the machine for APD are easily transportable, so that patients can leave home for a business journey or a vacation. A further advantage is that PD program does not need expensive investment or sophisticated resources and the overall cost of PD is lower than that of hemodialysis.

Some categories of patients benefit from PD for specific reasons, e.g. those without vascular access, those in which heparin adds risk of bleeding, those with autonomic insufficiency, in which fluid removal in the 4-hour time of a hemodialysis session causes severe hypotension. In addition, PD is strongly recommended as the dialysis of choice in children

Several conditions limit the use of PD. First of all, it is mandatory that patient and family members have adequate level of understanding, sense of responsibility and willingness to have active part in management of a life-threatening disease.

Abdominal surgery can generate peritoneal adhesions that obstacle distribution and emptying of peritoneal solution.

Protein loss is more consistent in PD than in hemodialysis (HD), so that PD is not advisable in malnourished patients.

In patients with large body surface area and high rates of metabolic waste production, depuration can be inadequate in spite of intensifying the number of cycles. The problem occurs mainly in anuric patients with no residual native renal function.

Adequacy of depurative efficacy of PD has to be regularly checked in order to prevent subtle retention of toxic products. A specific test has been designed named "peritoneal equilibration test", a simple and fast method to assess solute transport across the peritoneal membrane. In brief, the test measures the dynamics of the ratio of blood concentration over peritoneal fluid concentration of a product that diffuses across the peritoneal membrane (usually urea).

COMPLICATIONS OF PD

The two most important complications of PD are peritoneal infection and fibrosis.

Infection is a serious complication, associated with a significant risk for death. Infection of the exit site of the catheter is mostly caused by hand carrying Staphylococcus from the nostrils. Bacteria account for about 95% of infections, the rest are fungal. Nose sterilization can be obtained by local application of a gentamycin ointment. Hand contamination can be prevented by following standard disinfection protocols.

Symptoms of peritonitis in PD patients often are attenuated, consisting of abdominal tenderness and cloudy effluent, sometimes showing small fibrin clots. A leukocyte count higher than 100/μL in effluent fluid is diagnostic for inflammation. Note that inflammation does not mean necessarily infection and it may depend on hypersensivity to chemical components of dialysis fluid. Peritoneal fluid culture identifies the infective agent and addresses treatment through antibiogram.

Fibrosis is caused by repeated episodes of infection or as an incompatibility reaction that activates mesothelial cells inducing release of inflammatory and fibrogenic cytokines and growth factors. Paradoxically, a relevant pathogenic role is plaid by scatter factor, a growth factor that is committed to facilitate healing by inducing proliferation and movement of regenerated cells. In the setting of peritoneal dialysis cells made mobile are not tightly anchored to the peritoneal membrane and are washed away. Fibrosis is a cause of peritoneal dialysis failure and shifting to hemodialysis.

A dramatic form of fibrous thickening of peritoneum is sclerosing encapsulating peritonitis, that results from both visceral and parietal peritoneal inflammation. The cause of this complication is obscure and the only connected factor is a duration of PD longer than 5 years, which suggests a reaction to dialysis solution components.

ROLE OF PERITONEAL DIALYSIS AS RENAL REPLACEMENT TREATMENT

Today, approximately 15% of patients with terminal renal failure are treated with PD and the figure has been steady for many years. It is a minority and it seems that it will remain so for the future. Actually, the major limitation to its expansion is its same appealing reason, i.e. its management at home, that while allowing independence it places a great deal of responsibility on patients and their families.

A debated question is whether PD offers a different chance of survival and a different risk of morbidity compared with HD. Actually, there is no straightforward response. It is clear, in fact, that PD patients present bioincompatibility reactions, a chronic inflammatory state, a defective cell immunity similarly as HD patients. Thus, it seems that with some exceptions such as children or high surface adults, the choice of PD vs. HD should be decided by the patient.

CHAPTER 10

RENAL TRANSPLANTATION

The kidney was the first human organ to be transplanted successfully in 1954, but attempts to transplant parts of the body are reported in Ayurveda, an Indian textbook of medicine dating back to 2000 years B.C.E. It is intriguing that ancient transplant surgeons, not only Indian but also Byzantine were particularly skilled in transplanting the nose, having to replace the one excised from betrayers of the king or the king himself if he was dethroned.

In the absence of outcome reports we can assume that the results of these attempts were poor as it was of organs transplanted in animals and humans by European physicians from the 16th century onwards, until progress in Immunology shed light on the role of rejection of non-self as the cause of organ transplant failure.

Presently, renal transplant is the therapy of choice for terminal uremia and available data (2016) of the Global Donation and Transplantation Activity confirmed that the kidney ranks first among transplanted organs worldwide (around 80,000/year).

THE DONOR

There are three types of kidney donor: living, donor after brain death (DBD) and donor after circulatory death (DCD).

THE LIVING DONOR

Living donor is the preferred, for several reasons:

(i) Often donor and recipient are genetically related and share a major histocompatibility complex haplotype. Consequently, donor and recipient have at least 50% human leucocyte antigen (HLA) identical, a condition that reduces the risk for rejection.

(ii) The right moment to deliver transplantation can be tailored to recipient need, by-passing dialysis. Preemptive transplantation prevents dialysis related morbidities and enhances life expectancy.

(iii) Organ removal and grafting are strictly sequential, ischemia time is minimized and the risk for tubular necrosis and delayed graft function (DGF, see later) is reduced.

(iv) The donor can be thoroughly investigated to exclude transmittable diseases.

The number of transplants from living donors is growing to the point as to represent now more than 50% of all transplants in several countries.

DECEASED DONORS

After the concept of brain death and the criteria for its definition were universally accepted, deceased donors were exclusively dead-brain people in intensive care units where they received circulatory and respiratory support.

In the 1980s a shortage of brain-dead donors induced the consideration of procurement of kidney from circulatory dead people. Pilot programs in The Netherlands, U.K. and Spain demonstrated that kidneys recovered from DCD could work and programs of renal transplant from cardiac dead donors are now active in several countries. Improvement in perfusion technique before and after organ retrieval has significantly contributed to improve the quality of organs retrieved from DCD. Nonetheless kidneys from DCD have a higher prevalence of delayed graft function (DGF, see later) or primary non function. However, their long term survival is comparable to that of organs retrieved from DBD.

The obvious challenge of DCD donor is the long warm ischemia time lasting from cardiac arrest through resuscitation maneuvers to end of legal cardiac arrest. The latter varies in different countries, spanning from five minutes in The Netherland to twenty minutes in Italy, a very long time indeed, but yet compatible with functional recovery.

Actually, understanding whether a kidney retrieved from DCD has the chance for recovering is crucial. In our experience preimplantation biopsy is of help when it shows vascular necrosis of glomerular arterioles and tuft capillaries, that represent an ominous predictor of primary non-function. We find of little help attempts to stage tubular necrosis and interstitial edema and correlate their severity with graft outcome. Rather, a valuable method to predict success is perfusion of the excised kidney soon before implantation and measurement of resistance to flow. Perfusion devices and solutions designed just to perfuse the graft are now available and values of resistance lower than 0.4 are rarely wrong in predicting a graft's recovery.

In addition to being a thrust to using DCD, the dramatic discrepancy between the number of donors and patients waiting for a transplant has led to expanding the criteria that limit use of organ retrieved from DBD. So-called "expanded criteria donors" include over 60-year olds, or over 50-year olds with at least two of the following risk conditions: history of hypertension, serum creatinine greater than or equal to 1.5 mg/dL, death caused by vascular accident.

Kidneys retrieved from expanded donors would be biopsied to combine histological scoring and functional assessment in order to decide whether allocate the two kidneys singularly or as a "dual" transplant. On average the kidneys recovered from people at risk for cardiovascular disease have a lower quality, but they are worth being used for two reasons: first, their limited duration can be matched with recipient life expectancy, e.g. old donors and old recipients; second, the longer is time spent on hemodialysis, the shorter is the life expectancy. Interrupting dialysis, even for a few years, increases survival.

THE RECIPIENT

Any people with renal disease progressing to advanced renal failure should be informed of the possibility of having a transplant and should be invited to consider donation from a living donor before starting dialysis. The candidate to transplant should be taken in charge by a "Transplant Coordination" team of health professionals committed to implement diagnostic algorithms that state the feasibility of the transplant.

In brief, candidates to renal transplant would undergo two lines of investigation, one to detect clinical contraindications, the other one to define immunological profile.

Malignant tumors, active infections, severe organ failure, severe cardiovascular disease are the main obstacles to transplantation. Bladder and iliac vessels deserve special attention to exclude pathologies that hamper their anastomosis to the donor's ureter and renal vessels. Blood AB0 group, HLA typing, preformed anti-HLA antibodies are the basic immunological features that are explored. Age is no longer a limiting factor.

GRAFT ALLOCATION

Kidneys harvested for transplant are allocated according to algorithms that take into account major histocompatibility complex (MHC) compatibility, circulating preformed antibody, time spent on dialysis, age, and clinical conditions that represent a priority, e.g. lack of vascular access.

SURGICAL HINTS

The graft is placed in retroperitoneal space, heterotopic, i.e. in iliac fossa where its vessels are anastomosed with the recipient's Iliac vessels. Ureter of the graft is anastomosed to recipient's bladder. Native kidneys are left in place unless they are affected by a chronic infection that could be transmitted to graft or they are polycystic kidneys grown to huge dimension occupying so much space as to leave no place for the graft.

Bleeding, thrombosis, stenosis are possible complications of vascular surgery. A quite frequent problem is lymphocele, i.e. the collection of free lymphatic fluid in the retroperitoneal space. The abundancy of undrained lymphatic fluid and the resistance to stretching of the abdominal wall can generate a compression on the renal vessel or on the pelvis and cause acute renal failure.

A severe complication is acute ischemic necrosis of the ureter, that occurs when fine arterial vessels supplying the ureter are excised and there is no accessory vessel coming from the renal artery.

CAUSES OF GRAFT INJURY

No doubt that renal Transplantation is the best treatment for renal failure and no doubt that its outcome has a high rate of success, with 90% of grafts functioning after 5 years and 65% after 10 years. These encouraging figures, however, represent the result of a continuous struggle to repulse attacks that challenge graft survival. Apart from surgical complications, early injuries consist of insults caused by ischemia/reperfusion and rejection, that are later followed by renal toxicity of immunosuppressive drugs, chronic rejection, interstitial nephritis drug or virus dependent, relapse of primary disease, accelerated arteriosclerosis secondary to lipid and glucose dysmetabolism and hypertension.

DELAYED GRAFT FUNCTION AND PRIMARY NON FUNCTION

Seeing urine dropping out of a graft's ureter soon after graft vessels have been anastomosed is a moment of great satisfaction. Unfortunately, not all transplants work immediately, but about 30% of kidneys from DBD and 50% of kidneys from DCD start functioning after a time as long as to make it necessary post-transplant dialysis treatment. The condition is generically defined "delayed graft function" and it can be considered as the form of acute kidney injury (AKI) occurring in the graft. The feature that characterizes this AKI is that the damage induced by ischemia, mainly to tubular cells, is associated with a further inflammatory burst occurring when blood reperfused contacts endothelium. Actually, endothelium injured by ischemia expresses thrombogenic factors and release as cytokines and oxygen radicals that activate complement and attract leukocytes.

In most cases ischemia/reperfusion injury is reversible, but it leaves significant signs of its passage, consisting of interstitial fibrosis of variable extent. Furthermore, it increases the risk for acute rejection and shortens the expected survival of the graft.

PRIMARY NON-FUNCTION

This condition is the irreversible failure of the graft that does not even start functioning. It is either the consequence of a dramatic surgical complication, say thrombosis of vascular anastomosis, or the destructive assault of preformed anti-donor antibodies causing a hyperacute rejection.

ACUTE REJECTION

Acute rejection is the immune response of the recipient against non-self graft. Its frequency peaks in the first 6 months after transplantation, but it can occur at any time even after years. The powerful action of modern immunosuppressant drugs has changed its clinical presentation that in the past was synthetized by the triad of local pain, fever and urinary signs (oliguria, hematuria). A correspondence between these symptoms and biopsy proved acute rejection is now lower than 50%. Acute rejection is mainly suspected from a rise in serum creatinine level and is confirmed by renal biopsy. Biopsy-based staging of acute rejection (Banff classification) has been repeatedly revised and its description goes beyond the purpose of these lessons. In brief, it describes and quantifies the features of lesions caused by rejection to tubules, interstice arterioles and glomerular tuft. In most cases, acute rejection is cell-mediated and its typical lesion is tubulitis, i.e. infiltration of tubules by mononuclear cells that cross the tubular basement membrane. Vasculitis is signaled by adhesion of mononuclear cells to the endothelium of small arteries and arterioles and, in a progression of severity by neutrophil margination in peritubular capillaries, interstitial hemorrhage and fibrinoid necrosis of arteriole wall. Vasculitis indicates participation of humoral immunity in rejection pathogenesis.

HYPERACUTE REJECTION

This rejection is caused by preformed circulating antibodies against the donor that attack graft endothelium and cause a necrotizing thrombotic vasculitis. Prevention of such a dramatic event rests on "cross match", i.e. matching recipient serum with donor lymphocytes to detect antibody adhesion to lymphocyte and lymphocyte activation. Unfortunately the test can miss some antibodies directed against donor endothelial antigens that are not expressed on lymphocytes.

ACUTE LOSS OF GRAFT FUNCTION

Acute rejection is the most frequent , but not the unique cause of acute loss of graft function, an event that can occur at any time after transplantation. Apart from functional episodes due to volume depletion, vasoconstriction caused by excess calcineurin inhibitors is a reversible mechanism that would be prevented by regular control of blood trough levels but with exceptions, e.g.

when drug interference modifies pharmacokinetics. Calcineurin inhibitors can cause thrombotic microangiopathy that can be suspected by finding humoral indicators of hemolysis, low platelet count and schistocytes visible at microscopy in a blood smear. We have already mentioned lymphocele and urological obstruction. A very special cause of acute graft failure is interstitial nephritis caused by a virus of the polyoma family. The virus is present in the urinary tract of many healthy people as a non-pathogenic host, but immunosuppression makes it infective. Renal biopsy detects giant "decoy" tubular cells containing in nucleus viral particles in a scenario of interstitial infiltration of mononuclear cells and sometimes eosinophils. High blood level of viral DNA confirms the diagnosis.

CHRONIC TRANSPLANT NEPHROPATHY

Renal grafts can undergo a progressive loss of function associated with a fibrogenic process that involves all parts of the nephrons in a way that makes it difficult to recognize the various pathogenic components of the phenomenon. The process was described as "chronic transplant nephropathy" a tautologic definition that was eventually abandoned as traits specific for single etiopathogenic mechanisms could be identified. In fact, it is now possible to distinguish chronic rejection, i.e. immune mechanism, from chronic drug toxicity, the two major causes of chronic damage.

CHRONIC REJECTION

Chronic rejection was but a hypothesis until it was possible to detect in graft biopsy an indirect proof of antibody-mediated injury consisting of C4d fraction of complement bound to endothelium of peritubular capillaries and, less frequently, glomerular capillaries. C4d is a product of antibody-dependent complement activation that binds steadily to endothelium in contrast with antibodies that are cleaved away in a short time. As such, C4d is the memory of antibody mediated injury. Actually C4d by itself has no pathogenic role, but its relation with humoral rejection is supported by the detection of anti-donor circulating antibodies in patients in which C4d is expressed in renal tissue. Chronic rejection is also associated with a striking subendothelial fibrosis of small renal arteries, an impressive occlusive pathology leading to vessel obliteration and deposition of collagen in the tubular basement membrane in a multilayer stratification. A further sign of chronic rejection is transplant glomerulopathy, consisting of a visible thickening of the glomerular capillary wall, comparable in light microscopy to the picture of membranous nephropathy.

IMMUNOSUPPRESSIVE THERAPY

This concise section is not meant to present the topic of immune suppression in renal transplant, a complex expertise that belongs to nephrologists engaged in transplant program. We just wish to highlight the evolution of anti-rejection therapy and to discuss what benefits new therapies have produced.

In the early phase of renal transplantation, steroids were the only drug available to prevent and cure acute rejection. High boluses were delivered as induction therapy, then the dose was progressively but slowly tapered. Azathioprine was the first help to steroids and its main advantage was to permit lower doses of steroids and hence a reduction of steroid toxicity. This benefit, however, was attenuated by azathioprine's side effects, mainly its leukopenic action. Two major advances were the production of an antibody that blocked the CD25 molecule of interleukin-2 receptor (basiliximab) and the discovery of a fungal product that specifically inhibited T cell activity, cyclosporine.

Basiliximab proved excellent in defending the graft soon after its implantation with a highly favorable benefit/risk ratio, and became the cornerstone of induction therapy. Its use drastically reduced the incidence and severity of acute rejection in the early post-trasplant phase. Its limit was its failure in opposing humoral immunity, e.g. the assault of preformed anti-HLA and not anti-HLA anti-donor antibodies.

In the meantime, an alternative to azathioprine was made available, i.e mycophenolate, less toxic than azathioprine, but often causing gastrointestinal problems.

A further progress was the discovery on Easter Island (Rapa Nui in local language) of a soil bacteria product with antiproliferative immune suppressive effect. Rapamycine – the name reminds Rapa island – blocks lymphocyte response through a mechanism different from that of calcineurin inhibitors, so that it can be used in combination with them or as their substitute when they have to be discontinued because of severe renal toxicity. Actually, lack of renal toxicity is the most appreciable trait of rapamycine that otherwise has its own list of side effects, including slowing of tissue repair, lymphocele induction, platelet count decrease, bronchiolitis, gastrointestinal disturbances.

Belatacept, the last licensed immunosuppressant drug, raised great expectations because it was proved to be tolerogenic in experimental preclinical studies. Belatacept blocks the interaction between a couple of costimulatory molecules expressed on APC and lymphocytes, respectively, that is necessary for transducing antigen presentation by APC into lymphocyte activation. The transition of belatacept to human clinics has been quite disappointing because it does not induce tolerance, but it behaves as a moderately powerful immunosuppressant. Indeed, it is a possible alternative to traditional immunosuppressants, but with an important question mark represented by the rise in lymphoma incidence associated with its administration.

In summary, progress in immune suppressive therapy has changed the impact of acute rejection, that is now much less frequent and severe. The availability of different immunosuppressants with different mechanisms of action permits combinations that potentiate effectiveness while reducing side effects of single drugs. Inducing tolerance without compromising immune response to infective agents is still a dream.

DRUG TOXICITY

It is disappointing that the most effective drugs defending grafts against immune injury, i.e calcineurin inhibitors, such as cyclosporine and tacrolimus are toxic to the kidney to the point of being cause of graft failure. Cyclosporine has a dose dependent effect on glomerular hemodynamics consisting of a reversible increase in afferent arteriole resistance that causes a fall in glomerular plasma flow and in glomerular filtration rate. Long lasting persistent renal ischemia causes tubular atrophy and interstitial fibrosis. But ischemia is not the only nor the main fibrogenic mechanism of cyclosporine. Actually, cyclosporine disrupts the balance between fibrogenic and antfibrogenic factors changing their expression in renal tissue. Typical histopathological effects are a "striped" distribution of fibrosis, isometric vacuolization of cytoplasm of tubular cells and arteriolar hyalinosis. Protocol biopsies have shown that lesions caused by cyclosporine are present earlier than supposed and occur also when trough levels of the drug are in the right therapeutic range.

"Chronic transplant nephropathy" is no longer part of the Banff classification and in fact it is not a distinct nosographic entity. However, the term remains of some conceptual utility in that it underlies the mixture of pathogenic mechanisms that lead to late graft failure. Some of them are atherogenic, e.g. new onset diabetes, quite common after transplantation, hypertension, hyperlipidemia. Finally infections, and urinary tract obstruction play a part of variable importance.

INFECTIONS

Infections are a major complication of transplant, being facilitated by immunosuppression. Here we describe but the most frequent, in consideration of the possibility that any infective agent is potentially pathogenic in immune deficient people.

In the early post-transplant period, infections are mainly bacterial and related with surgery, while later virus and opportunistic agents prevail. The urinary tract is the most frequent site of bacterial infection and *E. Coli* is the most common infective culprit. Cytomegalovirus (CMV), a virus that causes a paucisymptomatic or flu-like infection in over 70% of the general population, belongs to the Herpes virus family and is the most important agent of viral infection in transplanted patients. In fact, immunosuppression permits reactivation of virus latent after primary infection, and raises its morbidity causing fever, gastrointestinal symptoms, liver enzyme increase, broncopneumonia as common effects. Similarly to CMV Epstein-Barr virus causes infection in 90% of the general population with variable symptoms, ranging from none to those of mononucleosis. In normal people primary infection is followed by protective immunization, but in immune-deficient patients it brings a high risk of inducing malignant B-lymphoproliferative disease. Therefore it is mandatory to exclude donations from anti-HBV antibody positive donors to recipients who are antibody negative.

Pseudocystis Carini is a yeast-like protozoan that causes interstitial pneumonia with fever, cough and dyspnea. Effective prevention is provided by trimethoprim-cotrimoxazole.

TAKE HOME MESSAGE

1. Dialysis is a life-saving replacement treatment delivered on average three 4-hour sessions weekly.
2. In Hemodialysis blood circulating in extracorporeal system contacts artificial material that activates leukocytes, coagulation and complement. Bioincompatibility reactions cause a chronic inflammatory state whose main pathogenic effect is cardiovascular damage.
3. Blood purification techniques consist of hemodialysis mainly based on solute clearance by diffusion , or hemofiltration based on convective transport. The two techniques can work together in hemodiafiltration.
4. Peritoneal dialysis is an alternative to hemodialysis delivered to 15% of patients on renal replacement treatment . It uses peritoneal membrane as dialysis filter.
5. Transplantation is the election therapy for chronic renal failure.
6. Major causes of late transplant failure are chronic rejection and drug toxicity.
7. Graft survival averages 70% at 10 years, in cadaver donor recipients.
8. Living donor transplantation gives the best chance of survival of recipient and graft.

REFERENCES

1. J. Himmelfarb, R.Vanholder, R.Mehrotra and M. Tonelli: The current and future landscape of dialysis. *Nature Reviews Nephrology* (2020). https://doi.org/10.1038/s41581-020-0315-4
2. N. Ngan, K.L. Lentine, A.X. Garg: Kidney Transplantation. *Nature Reviews Nephrology*, April 2017

SECTION 5

THE KIDNEY IN PREGNANCY

CHAPTER 11

PHYSIOLOGY OF THE KIDNEY IN PREGNANCY

Homer Smith, one of the founders of renal physiology wrote that "to a renal physiologist nothing is more interesting than a pregnant woman". Actually, pregnancy modifies many functions of the kidney and it is particularly intriguing that two of them are pivotal renal commitments, i.e. to ensure stability of extracellular fluid (ECF) volume and to autoregulate glomerular plasma flow and filtration rate. Indeed, these changes in renal function are part of a complex resetting of systemic hemodynamics and of hormonal regulatory systems that adapt to build up a new individual and to resist to the dramatic loss of blood that occurs at delivery.

EFFECTS OF PREGNANCY ON RENAL HANDLING OF SODIUM

It is impressive that the kidney, an organ that normally matches output of sodium to its intake and maintains constant sodium content in the body (and therefore ECF volume, see Chapter 1), during gestation retains about 900 mmol of sodium, corresponding to about 6.5 L of ECF volume. This retention of salt is the effect of a striking increase of aldosterone blood levels. It is noteworthy, however, that the increased distal tubular sodium reabsorption driven by aldosterone is contrasted by natriuretic adaptations, e.g. the rise in filtered sodium (see later), the rise in progesterone plasma levels, the release of prostaglandins E and in general the neurohumoral and hemodynamic responses that are activated by ECF volume expansion. Indeed, the prevalence of retention over loss is fragile to the point that pregnancy has been defined "a subtle salt-losing condition".

EFFECTS OF PREGNANCY ON GLOMERULAR HEMODYNAMICS

In the first weeks of gestation renal plasma flow increases sharply and rises to a maximum increment of about 60% at the second month, then remains high until delivery. Experimental micropuncture studies have shown that this change is the effect of a marked fall of afferent arteriole resistance. In addition to raising glomerular blood flow the dilatation of the afferent arteriole causes a rise in glomerular capillary hemodynamic pressure that increases ultrafiltration pressure. Therefore, the two determinants of ultrafiltration rate. i.e. the amount of plasma that is available for filtration and the pressure gradient that drives fluid through the filter contribute to raising the glomerular filtration rate, that in fact rises by 60%, a phenomenon that is unique in renal physiology.

RESETTING OF SYSTEMIC HEMODYNAMICS

Part of fluid retained in pregnancy is used to build the product of conception, part is distributed in the mother's body and expands ECF volume and its fraction represented by plasma. Such a relevant increase in plasma volume, however, is not associated with a rise in blood pressure (BP). Rather, BP decreases by 10-15 mm Hg due to a fall of the total peripheral resistances (TPR), a phenomenon that reflects the low sensibility of resistance vessels to angiotensin II (AII). Actually, IV infusion of angiotensin II in pregnant women raises BP much less than in non-pregnant, a phenomenon that depends on blunted vasoconstriction. Interestingly, women that are prone to developing pregnancy induced hypertension (PIH, see later) respond normally to AII, a behavior that has been proposed as a test predicting the onset of preeclampsia (Gant test).

EFFECTS OF PREGNANCY ON PLASMA OSMOLALITY

Plasma osmolality starts to decrease as early as after 3-4 weeks of gestation and attains a nadir of 10 mOsm around the 10th week that lasts till delivery. Plasma levels of vasopressin are normal and concentration/dilution of urine work perfectly.

URINARY TRACT IN PREGNANCY

Dilatation of the pelvis and ureters occurs in the last trimester in over 80% of pregnant women. The phenomenon is caused by the combination of compression by the growing uterus with relaxation of the muscular wall and reduced frequency of peristaltic contractions. Usually, the right ureter is more dilated than the left one because of its crossing over the dilated, tense right ovarian vein. The right hydroureter can cause pain during resting in bed that is relieved by changing position to the left side.

COAGULATION IN PREGNANCY

Pregnancy causes a resetting of hemostasis, coagulation and fibrinolysis that prompts an effective block of bleeding after delivery. Circulating levels of fibrinogen and factor VII increase progressively during gestation reaching a maximum at term, that consists of doubling of fibrinogen and ten times increase of factor VII.

The changes in the coagulation system, however are much more complex than a simple increase of levels of circulating procoagulant factors. Actually, inhibitors of coagulation such as protein S, antithrombin III and protein C and effectors of fibrinolysis like plasminogen increase too, so that the potentiation of coagulation is associated with a reduced stability of the system. Consequently, in pregnancy an imbalance between pro- and anticoagulant systems can undergo loss of control and cause catastrophic life-threatening disorders such as disseminated intravascular coagulation and cortical necrosis as discussed in the following chapter.

CHAPTER 12

RENAL DISORDERS AND PREGNANCY

PREGNANCY AND HYPERTENSION

The physiological adaptation of systemic hemodynamics occurring in pregnancy is disrupted in two pathological conditions characterized by arterial hypertension: pregnancy induced hypertension (PIH) and hypertension in pregnancy (HIP).

PREGNANCY INDUCED HYPERTENSION

PIH is a disorder exclusive to the human species that represents the leading cause of maternal death and an important cause of fetal morbidity. Its pathogenesis has been the object of a countless number of studies that have generated a plethoric number of hypotheses, but remains quite obscure. Epidemiology suggests a genetic substrate because women whose mother or sisters were affected are at higher risk for the disease. A high risk is associated with hypertension, chronic renal disease, systemic immune disorders in particular systemic lupus erythematosus (SLE) and antiphospholipid antibodies syndrome. Interestingly, the presence of fetus is not necessary for PIH development, as demonstrates its occurrence in women non-pregnant with vesicular mole.

The last finding indicates that the placenta is the site where the disease originates and in fact the earliest phenomenon observed consists of a defect in placentation that is followed by a systemic disorder of endothelium. The endothelial injury is visible in glomerular capillaries that present an "endotheliosis", i.e. swelling of endothelial cells. As premised, research has produced plenty of data on the mechanisms that activate the endothelium. We will not report in detail on this point, accepting as a matter of fact that endothelial dysfunction accounts for the symptoms of PIH.

In fact, activated endothelium releases endothelin, a powerful vasoconstrictor that raises total peripheral resistance and blood pressure. Endothelin is not the unique culprit for vasoconstriction, that results from a complex derangement of vasoactive agents including prostaglandins, angiotensin, nitric oxide and some identified more recently, e.g. soluble fms-like tyrosine kinase 1 (sFlt1), a circulating variant of vascular endothelial growth factor (VEGF) receptor (VEGFR) that blocks the trophic effect of VEGF on endothelial cells. Indeed hypertension occurs in a setting of hypovolemia that depends on increased permeability of peripheral capillaries and shifting of fluid to the interstice. Fluid redistribution contributes to generating peripheral edema, together with abundant proteinuria and hypoalbuminemia. Proteinuria is a major determinant of the clinical profile of the disease, whose former definition was EPH (Edema, Proteinuria, Hypertension) gestosis. The corresponding glomerular histopathological trait is endotheliosis, a swelling of endothelial cells often associated with deposition of a thin film of fibrin. In fact, injured endothelium activates hemostasis and coagulation. Low platelet count, fibrin deposition in the capillary wall, microthrombi and hemolysis revealed by helmet cells in blood smear, depict a scenario of thrombotic microangiopathy that can cause acute renal failure. A rare presentation of PIH is HELLP syndrome (acronym from Hemolysis Elevated Liver Enzymes Low Platelet), a combination of hemolysis, microangiopathy and liver injury. In the most dramatic cases disseminated intravascular coagulation

(DIC) occurs in which thrombosis and bleeding coexist in a life-threatening condition.

In summary, PIH is a systemic disease turned on by a defective placentation that causes activation of endothelium, new onset hypertension, proteinuria, edema, coagulation and hemostasis derangements and eventually convulsive attacks. The expression of symptoms is variable and improve after delivery.

DISSEMINATED INTRAVASCULAR COAGULATION (DIC)

DIC can be started by complications exclusive for gestation, including abruption placentae, septic abortion, intrauterine infection, amniotic fluid embolism, retained stillborn and uterine rupture. Furthermore, frank DIC can be the evolution of pregnancy induced hypertension. Symptoms include those caused by thrombosis as well as hemorrhage, that supervenes after massive activation of coagulation has consumed coagulation factors. Kidneys are inevitably targeted by DIC with variable severity from deposition of fibrin in glomerular capillaries and reversible acute renal failure to cortical necrosis, a catastrophic picture of tissue destruction with no possible recovery.

Diagnosis is supported by consumption of coagulation/hemostasis factors (low platelet, fibrinogen) and increased release of fibrin degradation products.

HEMOLYTIC UREMIC SYNDROME (HUS) IN PREGNANCY

Pregnancy associated HUS is a rare but severe complication occurring often in early post-delivery. It is an atypical form linked to variants of alternative complement pathway genes. Presentation is a dramatic picture of acute kidney injury that requires dialysis in 70% of patients and in 50% of cases is not reversible. Treatment consists of plasmapheresis, plasma infusion. Recurrence can occur in transplant patients.

CHRONIC HYPERTENSION IN PREGNANCY

This is the condition of women that are hypertensive and become pregnant. It is important to remember that in pregnancy blood pressure is lower by 15-20 mm Hg (systolic), 10-15 mm Hg (diastolic). Therefore, levels of blood pressure that would be considered moderate in non-pregnant people are highly pathogenic during gestation. In pregnant women hypertension causes ischemic injury to the placenta with poor growth of the fetus and premature birth of small for gestational age (SGA) babies. Furthermore, an injured placenta can affect endothelium and generate a PIH.

In pregnant women the physiological dilatation of the afferent arteriole blunts renal autoregulation that facilitates salt loss. In fact, experimental studies have shown that high perfusion pressure is transmitted to glomerular and postglomerular circulation, increasing GFR and reducing tubular sodium reabsorption. Accordingly, in women with chronic hypertension plasma volume has been found inversely related with blood pressure, a finding that suggests a defect of ECF volume caused by a derangement of normal sodium retention. In view of these findings any maneuver aimed to limit sodium gain, e.g. low salt diet or diuretic treatment should be avoided or reserved for life-threatening emergencies.

RENAL DISEASE AND PREGNANCY

Renal disease and pregnancy represent a reciprocal risk because renal disease is an obstacle to fetal growth and increases the risk for Pregnancy Induced Hypertension while pregnancy is often a booster that accelerates the progression to renal failure. Renal disease and pregnancy represent an association that can lead to serious maternal and fetal adverse effects. Counseling with experts is advisable to inform of the risks and plan an adequate check program.

EFFECTS OF PREGNANCY ON RENAL DISEASE

A woman with renal disease that becomes pregnant is at risk of accelerated loss of renal function during gestation. Retrospective studies have shown that the risk is very low in normotensive patients with mild reduction of GFR and low proteinuria but it increases as GFR decreases and it is particularly high in patients with nephrotic syndrome. Hypertension associated with renal disease is an independent risk factor for worsening of renal function.

EFFECTS OF RENAL DISEASE ON PREGNANCY

Woman with renal disease that conceive and do not stop gestation are at significant risk for adverse maternal and fetal outcomes. Risk increases as GFR decreases and peaks in patients on regular dialysis treatment, in whom conceiving is very rare, preterm delivery occurs in 90% of cases and 50% of fetuses die. About 25% of women with renal dysfunction develop preeclampsia, a figure that rises to 80% in hypertensive patients. In contrast with dialysis, renal transplant permits conceiving and pregnancy ending successfully in over 70%. Most of the medication necessary to prevent graft loss is not contraindicated in pregnant women, but some exceptions, e.g. mycophenolate and angiotensin converting enzyme (ACE) inhibitors exist.

URINARY TRACT INFECTION (UTI)

In pregnancy the pelvis and ureter dilate and peristaltic activity slows, mainly as an effect of high progesterone levels. In the last weeks of gestation an enlarged uterus can compress the pelvic tract of the ureter causing further dilatation of the urinary tract. These changes increase risk of diffusion of urinary infection from the bladder up to the pelvis. Acute pyelonephritis in a pregnant woman is an emergency, causing severe loin pain, high fever, vomiting and dehydration.

UTI in pregnancy is associated with relevant adverse effects, e.g. premature delivery, SGA babies, acute kidney injury and even fetal or maternal death. Therefore, it is current practice to treat any level of bacterial contamination in urine culture, rather than select only cases with a bacterial load higher than 100,000/mL.

TAKE HOME MESSAGE

1. Pregnancy is an extraordinary physiological condition, in which glomerular filtration rate and renal plasma flow increase by 50-60% and the kidneys reset sodium excretion to build up the product of conception and to expand maternal ECF volume.
2. Resetting of renal function in pregnancy is secondary to a marked fall of afferent arteriole resistance. This phenomenon impairs renal autoregulation and makes pregnancy a potential salt losing condition.
3. Pregnancy induced hypertension (PIH) is an exclusive disease of human gender, turned on by a placentation defect. Edema and proteinuria are associated symptoms. Eclamptic attacks, disseminated intravascular coagulation, HELLP syndrome are dramatic complications.
4. Renal disease and chronic hypertension increase the risk of PIH.

REFERENCES

1. A. Dal Canton: Renal hemodynamics in pregnancy, In VE Andreucci Editor, *The Kidney in pregnancy*, Martinus Nijoff. Publishing, pages 1-15, 1985
2. C.L. Sanders, J. Lucas: Renal disease in pregnancy. *Obstet Gynecol Clin North Am*: 28: 583-600, 2001

SECTION 6

DEGENERATIVE AND HEREDITARY RENAL DISORDERS

CHAPTER 13

RENAL CYSTIC DISORDERS

POLYCYSTIC KIDNEY DISEASE

This is an inherited autosomal dominant disease that can depend on a mutation in chromosome 16 (80% of cases) or in chromosome 4. The two proteins encoded by abnormal genes (Polycystin 1 and 2) are expressed in tubular cilium and form a calcium channel. The mutation disrupts cell growth and fluid transport resulting in proliferation of tubular cells that form cysts and inversion of planar cell polarity that causes fluid secretion into the cyst cavity.

Symptoms and progression of the disease are more severe in patients with altered chromosome 16 than in those affected in chromosome 4. In the former symptoms start earlier and renal failure makes replacement treatment necessary around the age of 50. Symptoms consist of pain in lumbar region either dull or colicky, episode of gross hematuria, associated with a bilateral palpable mass. Transformation of tubules into cysts is associated with a derangement in sodium reabsorption that causes polyuria, so that polycystic kidney disease is considered a salt losing nephropathy. With time, cyst growth can transform the kidneys into huge masses that displace the bowel and hamper diaphragm movement, causing constipation and shortness of breath. Cyst infection is not rare.

Furthermore, kidneys are not the unique target of the disorder, that is actually systemic and extrarenal localizations contribute symptoms and risks. The liver and pancreas are often involved in cyst formation, sometimes to the point of presenting organ failure. Aneurisms of cerebral arteries are a not frequent (less than 5%), but are a high-risk association.

Polycystic kidney disease (PKD) is easily recognized with an ultrasound investigation and when some doubt remains, possibly because of the early phase of the disease, a magnetic resonance or a CT scan are definitely diagnostic.

Interestingly, the inherited nature of APKD has not discouraged attempts to stop its progression to renal failure. A three-year treatment with tolvaptan, a vasopressin antagonist, vs. placebo reduced the rate of GFR loss, but caused important adverse effects. Enlargement of the kidney and liver was slower in patients treated with octreotide, a long acting analogue of somatostatin, the inhibitor of growth hormone.

The surrogate nature of primary outcomes and the relevance of side effects are limiting the implementation of these treatment in clinical practice.

MEDULLARY CYSTIC DISEASE/ NEPHRONOPHTHISIS

These diseases are inherited and share similar histopathological findings but they differ in inherited pattern, that is autosomal dominant in medullary cystic disease (MCD), autosomal recessive in nephronophthisis (NPT). In addition, MCD is an adult disease while NPT can occur in children. Small cysts are located in the medulla mainly close to the cortical border. Renal histopathology shows tubular atrophy and interstitial fibrosis progressing to renal scarring. Symptoms are variable, from cases in which the disease is silent and is discovered after occasional detection of altered serum creatinine values to a salt-losing picture or a complex systemic disorder involving eye (NPT and retinitis pigmentosa) in Senior-Loken syndrome, or central nervous system (NPT and cerebellar ataxia) in Joubert syndrome. In some adults with MCD hyperuricemia independent of renal failure can occur.

SIMPLE RENAL CYSTS

Ultrasound abdominal investigation often detects asymptomatic renal cysts that can be solitary or multiple and in the latter case are often bilateral. These "simple renal cysts" can deform the adjacent parenchyma, but do not alter the structure of the kidney. They are often exophytic and represent a benign degeneration, whose prevalence increases with age, up to more than 50% in males over 70. Simple cysts can grow up to 10 cm diameter and cause tenderness of the loin. Anecdotal cases of cysts causing hypertension, urinary obstruction or abdominal emergency due to rupture are reported, but no significant relation between simple cysts and any clinical manifestation has been found in a large epidemiological study performed on more than 15,000 people sampled from the general adult population.

SPONGE KIDNEY

Sponge kidney is a congenital disease that becomes symptomatic in adulthood. Family clustering of some cases has suggested an inherited transmission, but in contrast with this hypothesis the disease can be unilateral. It is supposed that the disease depends on a defect in renal embryogenesis, i.e. in the interaction between the ureteric bud and the metanephric mesenchyme. Sponge kidney is not properly a cystic disease, but a malformation of the Bellini ducts that present pseudocystic dilatations. These "pockets" facilitate formation of stones, mostly containing calcium that makes them visible in a plain abdomen radiography. The regular disposition of the stones forming a semicircular figure interrupted medially in correspondence of the pelvis opening is diagnostic. Symptoms and evolution are those of renal stones. The pseudocysts that form a template for stones are open into duct lumen so that stones often move in the urinary tract and cause pain, hematuria and obstruction.

CHAPTER 14

HEREDITARY NON-CYSTIC RENAL DISORDERS

INHERITED GLOMERULOPATHIES

ALPORT SYNDROME

Alport syndrome is an inherited disease that affects the kidneys and other organs, among which the inner ear and eye are those that represent the classic form. The disorder is caused by different pathogenic mutations located in 3 genes coding for type IV collagen, *COL4A3*, *COL4A4* and *COL4A5*. Type IV collagen forms basal membranes and is expressed in several organs. The variety of mutations accounts for variations in organs involved and clinical presentation, as well as for genetic mode of transmission, that can be X-linked (gene *COL4A5*) or autosomal recessive (genes *COL4A4* and *COLA4A3*).

In the majority of cases renal symptoms start in late childhood or early adult age and consist of episodes of gross hematuria or abnormal findings in urine analysis (microscopic hematuria, proteinuria). Hypertension and loss of renal function appear later as the disease progresses to renal failure. Progression leads 50% of patients with X-linked form to dialysis or transplantation at the age of twenty-five. In other forms the rate of progression is not as predictable, but usually slower. Loss of hearing affects high frequency sounds and parallels renal symptoms. Renal histology shows splitting of glomerular capillary basement membrane and mesangial matrix expansion eventually resulting in glomerulosclerosis. The eye is affected in 25% of cases and the part involved is the lens that has a cone shape (lenticonus). In a few cases, yellowish/whitish flakes are visible in the retina, with no interference with visus.

NON-MUSCLE MYOSIN IIA GENE MUTATION

A clinical picture similar to Alport syndrome is caused by autosomal dominant mutations of gene encoding for heavy chain 9 of non-muscle myosin II. As yet 35 mutations of the gene have been identified that are characterized by a low platelet count and giant platelets. Only some mutations cause renal symptoms either alone or associated with hearing impairment and cataract. In addition to huge platelets as large as red blood cells, blood smear shows cytoplasmic inclusions in neutrophils. The variable shape and dimension of these inclusions formed by aggregated myosin molecules have been considered specific features of distinct entities (Sebastian syndrome, Flechtner syndrome, Dohle bodies in May-Hegglin anomaly) but whether their different morphology has any pathogenic impact is unknown. Easy bruising and hematomas are the consequence of low platelet count, but spontaneous bleeding is rarely severe. However, the risk of hemorrhage is associated with surgery, delivery and trauma. Proteinuria and microscopic hematuria are urinary symptoms that express the renal involvement, consisting of progressive glomerulosclerosis.

THIN GLOMERULAR BASEMENT MEMBRANE DISEASE

This is an autosomal dominant condition that causes hematuria. Episodes of gross hematuria remit by themselves without any additional symptom, nor any loss of renal function. Microscopic hematuria and low grade proteinuria are currently found. Diagnosis rests on renal biopsy showing at electron microscopy a thinned glomerular capillary basement membrane, less than 240 nm thick. Indeed, the condition is not really a disease since it does not affect renal function, but it has to be considered in differential diagnosis of clinical settings presenting recurrent macroscopic hematuria.

FABRY DISEASE

Fabry disease is an X-linked disorder caused by a defect of gene coding for alpha-galactosidase, an enzyme that breaks down glycosphingolipids. Shortage of the enzyme causes lipid accumulation in lysosomes. In the kidney, lipid engorgement occurs particularly in cells of blood vessels, but also in tubular cells and podocytes. The disease is systemic and other tissues affected that give rise to major symptoms are myocardium, nerves and skin. Symptoms occur in both sexes but are much more severe in males in most of whom, in the absence of treatment, renal failure makes it necessary to replace renal function within the age of 40. Renal presentation includes in some patients nephrotic syndrome. Skin lesions consist of angiocheratoma corporis diffusum, i.e. purple-bluish spots formed by dilated capillaries in sclerotic skin frame typically located in the buttocks and genital area. Heart involvement is common, reflecting lipid accumulation in all cardiac structures and is the cause of death in over 50% of patients. Burning pain of hands and feet is a tearing symptom of peripheral neuropathy. Early diagnosis is extremely important because the enzyme alpha-galactosidase is now available for substitutive therapy that can prevent progression of organ damage.

GENETIC DISORDERS OF PODOCYTES

Podocytes are glomerular cells planted on the outer side of the glomerular basement membrane that represent the main barrier to protein filtration into Bowman's space. Inherited disorders of podocytes cause abundant proteinuria and nephrotic syndrome.

Autosomal recessive mutations of genes coding for podocin and nephrin, two transmembrane proteins expressed in the slit diaphragm, cause nephrotic syndrome in children. Indeed, nephrin related disease starts before birth and has a dramatically accelerated course that sometimes requires immediate post-birth dialysis. The condition is known as Finnish type congenital nephrotic syndrome, because the first cases were described in Finland. Podocin related disease starts later, usually within the first years of life, but in some heterozygous cases it occurs in adulthood. Besides mutations of nephrin and podocin genes, rare cases of glomerulosclerosis dependent on mutations of other podocyte genes have been acknowledged in adults. These genes code for proteins that link nephrin and podocin with a kinase (*CD2AP*), regulate actin expression (*ACTN4* and *INF2*) or calcium transport (*TRPC6*). No doubt that the family is destined to be enriched with new entries.

GENETIC TUBULAR DISORDERS

In view of the complexity of functions operated by the tubule and of the plenty of proteins that regulate tubular transport, transmembrane exchange and fluid flows, the number of disorders dependent on defects of gene coding for tubular proteins seems really limited.

Tubular acidosis has been already described in Chapter 4. Here we describe inherited disorders of tubular handling of aminoacid, glucose, phosphate and sodium.

AMINOACIDURIA

Circulating aminoacids are freely filtered and normally are completely recovered by active transporters. Groups of affine aminoacids use the same transporter, so that a defective transporter causes loss of several aminoacids. However, a single aminoacid in a group can account for clinical effects.

CYSTINURIA

Cystinuria is due to a mutation of basic amino acid transporter, that causes urinary wasting of cystine, lysine, ornithine and arginine. Cystine is pathogenic because of its low solubility in urine at low pH, that causes crystal precipitation and stone formation. Colicky pain, obstruction, infection and in general symptoms and complications of urinary stones start in early adult age. The disease has a prevalence of 1:7,000 in general Western population, that rises to 1:2,500 in Libyan Jews. Cystine hexagonal translucent crystals are easily identifiable in urinary sediment, while stones can be missed at plain abdomen X-ray because of their X-ray transparency. A rotten egg smell can be smelt in the urine. Diet limiting cystine intake and stabilization of urinary pH around neuter or moderately basic values are effective in preventing stone formation.

DEFECTIVE NEUTRAL AMINOACID TRANSPORT (HARTNUP DISEASE)

Thirteen neutral aminoacids are eliminated in excess in urine, but symptoms depend on loss of one, e.g. tryptophan that is an internal source of nicotinamide, known also as vitamin B_3. Deficiency of tryptophan derived vitamin, when not compensated by increased alimentary intake, causes a skin rash that reproduces that of pellagra. Additional symptoms are neurological (intention tremor, hallucinations, unsteady gait) and gastrointestinal (diarrhea, malabsorption). Integration of intake (50 to 300 mg/day) to prevent symptoms is rationale.

FANCONI SYNDROME

Aminaciduria is a feature of Fanconi syndrome as part of a generalized disorder of proximal tubular reabsorption, that also causes loss of bicarbonate, phosphate, glucose, sodium, potassium, uric acid. The tubular defect can be inherited or acquired. The most frequent inherited form is cystinosis, a rare storage disease due to an enzymatic defect that causes lysosomal accumulation of the aminoacid cystine. Acquired forms depend on tubular cell injury caused by heavy metal poisoning, e.g. lead, drugs (aminoglycoside antibiotics, expired tetracycline), or tubulointerstitial nephritis.

Symptoms reflect impaired availability of substances lost in urine. Hypophosphatemia causes rickets in children and osteomalacia in adults. Aminoacid, glucose and phosphate shortage cause malnutrition and failure to thrive. Bicarbonaturia generates type II metabolic acidosis. Replacing sodium can be difficult by increasing sodium intake, so that most patients with Fanconi syndrome have a chronic depletion of ECF volume, responsible for hypotension, fatigue and thirst. Increased sodium delivery to the distal tubule raises the exchange of sodium for potassium and causes hypokalemia.

DISORDERS OF SODIUM REABSORPTION

Bartter syndrome

This syndrome includes core symptoms, i.e. natriuresis, hypotension, metabolic alkalosis and hypokalemia that result from an inherited defect of sodium reabsorption in the thick segment of Henle's ascending limb. In this tubular segment sodium reabsorption is operated by the coordinated activity of NKCC2 cotransporter, Na^+/K^+-ATPase pump, chloride channel ClC-Kb and ROMK potassium channel.

NKCC2 is expressed in the luminal membrane and transfers one sodium one potassium and two chloride ions from the lumen into the cell. The Na^+ ions are then pumped out of the cell through the basolateral membrane by the Na/K^+-ATPase pump. The Cl^- ions move out through the basolateral voltage gated Cl^- channel ClC-Kb, while excess K^+ crosses the apical membrane through the ROMK channel. A defect in any of these mechanisms inhibits Na^+ reabsorption and causes core symptoms of Bartter syndrome but with different severity and additional specific features. Detailed description of various types of Bartter syndrome is beyond the scope of the present handbook. However, we feel it important to point out that infantile forms are more severe than adult ones.

All forms are rare, the most frequent being the so called "classic" one that depends on defective NKCC2, is transmitted as recessive autosomic trait and replicates the effects of furosemide.

Gitelman syndrome

Gitelman syndrome is an autonomic recessive disease caused by a genetic defect of the NaCl cotransporter NCC expressed in the apical membrane of distal tubular cells. NCC is the target of thiazide diuretics and symptoms are similar to those caused by the drug, first of all sodium wasting and related effects on extracellular fluid volume, i.e. hypotension, muscle cramps, thirst, dizziness, drop attacks. Symptoms start mostly in children, but in a minority are delayed to early adult age. Hypomagnesemia and hypocalciuria reflect the impact of altered intracellular Na and Cl concentrations on activity of Ca/Mg channel TRPV5 expressed in the luminal membrane and of NCX countertransport that exchanges Ca^{++} for Na^{+} in the basolateral side.

TAKE HOME MESSAGE

1. Simple renal cysts are degenerative formations whose prevalence increases with age. Pathological effects are rare. Anecdotal hypertension, pain, infection, have been reported.
2. Adult polycystic kidney disease is the most frequent renal cystic disease. Inherited as dominant trait, there are two types, type 1 is the worse one.

REFERENCES

1. M. Bisceglia, C. Galliani, C. Senger, C. Stallone, A. Sessa: Renal cystic disease: a review. *Adv Anat Pathol*: 13: 26-56, 2006
2. L. Mehta, B. Jim: Hereditary Renal Diseases. *Semin Nephrol*: 37:354-361, 2017

APPENDICES

APPENDIX 1

DISORDERS OF URINARY APPARATUS

In this Appendix we describe two disorders whose principal localization is the urinary tract, i.e. the conduits that drive urine out, but that can extend to the kidney: infections and stones. Indeed, they are disorders of the urinary apparatus that often bring the patient to the operating room. Acknowledging the two sides of this issue we present it as an appendix of our *Textbook of Nephrology* and address the reader to texts of Urology for the parts that are about surgical competence.

URINARY TRACT INFECTIONS

Bacterial infections of urinary tract (UTIs) are very frequent in general population and occur at any age in both sexes, but short urethra, physical stress during sexual activity and pregnancy account for a higher prevalence in females. Malformations, stones, obstruction, diabetes, neurogenic bladder, prostate hypertrophy, urinary catheterization are conditions that increase the risk for UTIs.

ETIOPATHOGENESIS

Most of UTIs are ascending, i.e. are caused by bacteria that enter into the urethra from adjacent skin, then spread proximally. Most of the bacteria originate from rectal flora such as *Escherichia Coli*, that accounts for 80% of community acquired infections. Other common infective bacteria are *Proteus, Klebsiella, Pseudomonas, Enterococci*. UTIs represent 50% of hospital acquired infections, 40% of which are associated with urinary catheterization. Common bacterial species that cause UTIs succeed in invading the uroepithelium thanks to the expression of superficial molecules named adhesins that permit their anchorage to epithelial receptors, so that they resist to mechanical washing from urinary flow. Furthermore, once planted in the epithelium, bacteria organize a biofilm that forms a protective barrier against immune attacks.

ACUTE UTIs

Clinical presentation of UTIs depends on the site of urinary tract involved and on the state of the host, i.e. on factors that "complicate" the infection. Complicated UTIs are those that occur in patients that present any condition that facilitates urinary infection or hinders its healing. Urethritis causes urgency dysuria pollakiuria. Bladder infection (cystitis) reproduces the symptoms of urethritis with the addition of tenesmus and in severe cases fever, gross hematuria, pyuria. Localization to the pelvis generally does not spare the kidney (pyelonephritis, see later). Acute pyelonephritis is a severe disorder characterized by high fever, loin pain reactive to finger pressure in the costovertebral angle, fever arising with chills, nausea and vomiting and a prostrating malaise. In elderly people, immunodeficient patients and patients with severe comorbidities, pyelonephritis is a life-threatening condition.

RECURRENT UTIs

Recurrence of UTI is frequent, especially in women, either as relapse or reinfection. Relapse is the reappearance of symptoms after a period of remission that was not real healing. In relapse, bacteria are not fully eradicated and start reproducing as the antibiotic is withdrawn. Urine culture detects the same pathogen found before starting treatment. In general, relapse is the expression of conditions that protect pathogens or impair therapeutic efficiency causing incomplete sterilization of urine, such as indwelling catheters, urine retention in the bladder due to prostatic hypertrophy, diverticula, malformation, uterine prolapse.

In general, reinfection is caused by circumstances that facilitate entry of pathogens into the urinary tract, rather than by its intrinsic defects. A typical circumstance is cystitis that follows sexual activity in women, or in both sexes bowel disturbances, or intake of food that causes pelvic congestion, e.g. chili pepper.

Relapsing infections are difficult to stop unless one eliminates the predisposing condition. Guidelines suggest to cure recurrent urinary infections, defined as two episodes or more in 6 months, or three episodes or more in one year, with "continued prophylaxis", that consists of prescribing antibiotics for a long time, at least 6 months.

CHRONIC UTIs

Chronic UTIs are the continuation of acute infections that do not heal because of the presence of one or more conditions that are an obstacle to urine sterilization. Symptoms are similar to those of acute infection, but attenuated. This is the case of chronic pyelonephritis, whose most common symptoms include lumbar tenderness, low grade fever, cloudy urine, urine smelling of ammonia. Urinary analysis discloses proteinuria, microscopic hematuria, leukocytes. Urinary pH is often alkaline when the bacterial pathogen produces urease, the enzyme that converts urea to ammonia. The disease is unilateral in the majority of cases and causes a progressive decrease of renal size and an irregular contour due to retracting scars. Histology shows interstitial fibrosis and infiltration of inflammatory cells, tubular atrophy and variable tubular dilatation. Dilated tubules contain amorphous proteinaceous material stained by eosin and at first glance look like thyroid follicles. Periglomerular fibrosis and glomerular sclerosis occur in the late stage of disease. Eventually the inflammatory activity gives up as tissue scarring progresses leading to shrinkage of the organ.

The pyelonephritic "shrunken" kidney, however can remain a source of morbidity as the cause of hypertension.

Sodium wasting and related effects on extracellular fluid volume, i.e. hypotension, muscle cramps, thirst, dizziness, drop attacks. Symptoms start mostly in children, but in a minority are delayed to early adult age. Hypomagnesemia and hypocalciuria reflect the impact of altered intracellular Na and Cl concentrations on activity of Ca/Mg channel

URINARY STONES

Urinary stones are one of the most common disorders occurring in the general population. Their prevalence is maximal in adult males, but they form at any age and independently of sex or race. Cross sectional prevalence in the general population is around 5%, but life time prevalence is three times higher. Furthermore, recurrence rate approximates 10%/year and jumps to 70% over a 20 year period.

Etiopathogenesis

Stone formation starts with nucleation, i.e. precipitation of salt or organic products that generate a "nucleus" over which stone matter progressively stratifies. Most often the nucleus is made of crystals, but it can be amorphous. The nucleus can aggregate components different from itself. The common mechanism that causes precipitation is a concentration of material higher than it can be dissolved. The phenomenon, named supersaturation, depends on the volume of solvent, on the load of solute produced and filtered or secreted, on pH and on the presence of substances that increase the solubility of the material. A further pathogenic factor is the regularity of urine flow that can be disrupted by malformations or obstruction. A particular form of nucleation is represented by Randall's plaques that are the progenitors of stones of calcium oxalate. The plaques are concretions that form in the interstice of papilla, grow by aggregation and eventually break the wall of Bellini ducts and continue to grow in the urinary conduit.

Clinical presentation

Stones evoke a typical colicky pain caused by spastic contraction of the pelvis or ureter, a reaction that usually occurs when the stone is displaced by urine flow and peristalsis along the urinary tract. Pain is excruciating and spreads down to the testis or labia. Large stones that are too big to move, especially those that occupy the pelvis cause a dull pain in the costal vertebral angle that is intensified by finger pressing. Hematuria is present in microscopic form in almost all patients and gross hematuria is common.

Obstruction is a major complication that can cause renal damage disproportionate to its symptoms. In fact, it not rare to find a hydronephrotic kidney in asymptomatic patients. The case can occur for example, when a colicky episode due to a ureteral stone stops spontaneously and is not followed by investigation aimed to localize the stone. Prolonged obstruction that stops urine flow causes progressive atrophy of renal tissue.

Stone composition

The most common stones are made of calcium salts, in particular calcium phosphate and calcium oxalate. Idiopathic hypercalciuria, defined as urinary daily calcium excretion >270 mg/24 h in men and >240 mg/24 h in women is the main mechanism leading to calcium stone formation. Idiopathic hypercalciuria can be absorbitive, i.e. dependent on excess intestinal calcium absorption, or on renal calcium leakage. Secondary hypercalciuria can result from primary hyperparathyroidism and various disorders that cause hypercalcemia, i.e. excess vitamin D_3 intake or endogenous vitamin D_3 release (sarcoidosis), excess calcium intake (milk-alkali syndrome), or from diseases that mobilize calcium from bone (chronic acidosis, bone invasion by neoplasms). Calcium stones are radio-opaque and visible on a plain X-ray. Stones of calcium oxalate are hard, present an irregular shape with sharp prominences and are black or dark brown. Crystals visible in urinary sediment are prismatic, looking like diamonds. Stones of calcium phosphate are smooth, yellowish or pale gray. After calcium stones, urate stones rank third in frequency. Uric acid is the product of purine metabolism and its urinary excretion depends on endogenous production and on the intake of purine with food. On average daily uric acid excretion is 700-800 mg. Diets rich in red meat, fish, organ meat like liver contain high amounts of purine and increase urinary uric acid load and risk for crystal precipitation. Other conditions that increase uricosuria are drugs, e.g. salicylic acid, indomethacin, losartan and tumor lysis due to chemotherapy. However, the most important determinant of uric acid supersaturation is urine acidity that markedly reduces uric acid solubility when pH <5.5.

Special stones are those that form in alkaline urine infected with bacteria that produce urease, the enzyme that hydrolyzes urea to ammonium and CO_2. The combination of ammonium with phosphate and magnesium gives rise to Struvite a mineral whose crystals are described as reproducing the shape of the cover of a coffin. Struvite stones are Rx opaque and often completely fill the pelvis and calyces forming a cast that resembles the horns of a stag.

As described in chapter 15, inherited cystinuria, a tubular defect that blocks reabsorption of amino acid cystine, is associated with precipitation of typical exagonal crystals and stones.

Diagnosis

Ultrasound is the investigation of choice, showing the typical shadow cone. However, an echography can miss small stones in the ureter or in the bladder, that can be detected by a CT scan. The chemical composition is often recognized by the shape, color, hardness and form of crystals in urinary sediment.

Therapy

In the past, surgery was the only means to remove a stone. Now instrumental procedures allow less invasive interventions that strongly reduce the therapeutic place for traditional surgery. We address to urology texts for approaching this item.

Prevention has maximal importance, especially secondary ones in view of the very high number of recurrences. Diluting urine by drinking is the first and main way to prevent supersaturation, a purpose that is contributed by dietary regimens limiting intake of stone forming matter. Finally, maximal solubility has to be targeted by adjusting urine pH and delivering compounds, e.g. citrate, that are acknowledged for having the property of increasing the amount of calcium salts that can be found in a given volume of water.

BOX 1 Rare stones

It was perhaps forty years ago. The teenager was a skinny girl with pale-blue eyes, and a timid but capturing smile. She lived with her family in a remote small village in a mountain region, about 1,000 m over sea level, about 70 km far from the nearest town.

The girl was admitted to the General Hospital after recurrency of abdominal colicky pain had become so frequent as to hamper school attendance. No doubt that pain was due to renal stones, she had collected many of them. Their aspect was unusual, they were 3-7 mm large, dark grey, scale-like and quite friable. I was just graded M.D. and I was training at the General Hospital with Mino a very good friend of mine and collegue from middle School to University. The "case" gained our attention after that all exams programed to diagnose a stone disorder missed the scope: normal plain X-ray of abdomen, within normal limits serum calcium, phosphate, uric acid and urinary excretion of calcium, phosphate, urate, oxalate and citrate. Furthermore chemical analysis of the stones made in the Hospital lab did not succeed in defining their composition and the stones were sent to the Department of Physics for spectrometric analysis, whose result was astonishing: the main component was a zinc salt! Mino and I were overexcited for what seemed to be an exceptional finding and spent the next two days in the Hospital library reading thousands of Current Contents, weekly reports of papers published in the broad area of Life Sciences, a tearing and time consuming way to update research findings, but the only one available in the pre-internet era. Two days later, re-entering in the ward we soon met our tutor and informed him of our unsuccessful exploration. As we were describing our bibliographic efforts, the tutor seemed amused and at the end of our tale he said: "so, you are the only ones that do not know the story!"

→

The story was that the girl had a new colicky attack and a nurse checking for girl's state and not finding her in bed, looked for her in the toilet... just in time to find her putting stones in the urine vessel.
The confession was complete. The girl was not happy with school which was 1 hour from home, and with waking up early in winter in a chilly house where heating was provided by old coal stoves. And the stove was the source of stones, or better the tin chimney that discharged the smoke outside. The pipe was painted with a silvery stain containing zinc, and every year a new paint layer was painted over the old one, creating a thick crust from which fragments were easily detached and used as stones.
Stones were the masterpiece of girl's tricky representation because they proved that pain was not an invention.
And the end? A college in the town.

APPENDIX 2

CORRECT USE OF DIURETICS

Diuretics are drugs that increase urinary output by inhibiting tubular sodium and water reabsorption. Actually, they induce an osmotic diuresis because water is passively dragged by sodium. Being drugs that deplete body sodium, all diuretics decrease ECF volume. In clinical practice diuretics used are thiazides, high-ceiling diuretics, potassium sparing diuretics and aldosterone inhibitors.

Thiazides are hydrochlorothiazide and chlorthalidone. Both have limited power and do not work when GFR is lower than 40-50 mL/min. Furthermore, the range of the dose dependent effect is narrow, e.g. the maximum effect of chlortalidone is obtained with a 50 mg dose, vs. a minimum dose of 25 mg. Today thiazides are used mainly in combination with antihypertensive drugs, especially ACE-inhibitors. Their antihypertensive effect reaches a maximum after 3-4 weeks. Interestingly, for the first 1-2 weeks after starting treatment the initial decrease in blood pressure is caused by hypovolemia but later blood volume normalizes and total peripheral resistances (TPR) decrease. This conversion is held as an indirect demonstration that Guyton's hypothesis on the pathogenesis of essential hypertension is correct. Guyton elaborated a model in which essential hypertension starts as the effect of a constitutive hypervolemia and transforms with time in a TPR dependent effect. The rise in TPR would be a response to peripheral tissue hyperperfusion.

High-ceiling diuretics are furosemide, bumetanide, torasemide and ethacrynic acid, but in practice furosemide is the one used in the overwhelming majority of cases. The definition "high-ceiling" refers to the high dose range in which dose and diuretic effect are incremental. They are very powerful and at high dose they also work in patients with very low GFR.

The high power of furosemide is associated with the rapid onset of action and brisk activity peaking in 2-3 hours. Furthermore, it can be injected. The combination of pharmacokinetic and pharmacodynamic features of furosemide make it invaluable in an emergency, e.g. acute heart failure, or in cases of renal failure. Of course, to benefit from the characteristics of furosemide, one has to exploit its "high-ceiling" property. For example, to treat a patient with low GFR (say 20 mL/min) furosemide has to be delivered in single bolus of 250-500 mg, rather than split in multiple small doses, none of which would be effective. In addition, furosemide is overused in patients in which chlortalidone should be the diuretic of choice. We mean patients with normal renal function that are hypertensive or have peripheral edema in the absence of critical symptoms. Due to its brisk action furosemide extracts fluid from circulation in two-three hours, a time too short to permit refilling, during which hypovolemia can cause hypotension, faintness or collapse. In contrast, chlortalidone splices its diuretic action in 24 hours, permitting vascular refilling and protecting from effects of hypovolemia.

Furosemide and thiazides increase the delivery of sodium to the last part of distal tubule and cortical collecting duct.

In these tubular segments principal cells reabsorb a quite constant fraction of sodium delivered, exchanging it for potassium.

This loss of potassium is inhibited by so-called potassium sparing diuretics and by aldosterone antagonists. Amiloride and triamterene regulate passage of sodium from the lumen into distal tubular cells and collecting duct cells by closing sodium channels.

The resulting accumulation of sodium in the lumen impairs the electrochemical gradient that drives potassium from the cell to the lumen. Consequently less potassium is excreted. Of course the efficacy of these drugs depends on the amount of sodium that is left in the lumen and this, in turn, on sodium delivery. For this reason these diuretics are particularly efficient in sparing potassum when they are associated with diuretics that inhibit sodium reabsorbtion in tubular segment proximal to their site of action. Aldosterone antagonists similarly reduce sodium passage through sodium channels by decreasing the number of channels. It is useless to say that for being effective serum aldosterone concentration must be elevated.

APPENDIX 3

GLOBALIZATION, MIGRATION AND RENAL DISEASES

Travel facilities, economical globalization and migration of people forced to leave their native country because of famine, war, persecution or desire to improve their life style is a global phenomenon whose dimension is underestimated because many are illegal immigrants. Most immigrants come from poor underdeveloped countries where environmental and hygienic conditions are a high risk for infectious and parasitic transmittable diseases.

The other side of the coin is represented by people of affluent countries that move abroad for business or tourism and develop parasitic or infectious diseases. In all these conditions diagnosis can be missed because it is not even considered. Aim of this appendix is far from describing all possible diseases that can be imported by moving people, rather it is to present but a few examples of diseases that are poorly considered in differential diagnosis in developed Countries, because there is not enough awareness of how much there epidemiology is changing.

TUBERCULOSIS (TBC)

Tuberculosis is not a migration disease, but presently its incidence in Western countries is mainly sustained either by people who have migrated from Africa or South Eastern Asia, where it is the first infectious cause of death, or by HIV positive people. The 2019 tuberculosis surveillance and monitoring in Europe Report has confirmed the high prevalence of multidrug resistance in European TBC cases. As for diagnosis, prophylaxis and therapy, we address the reader to specialized sources of information.

SCHISTOSOMIASIS

Schistosomiasis is a parasitic disease caused by worms of the genus *Schistosoma*. Humans are infected by larvae hosted in freshwater snails that spread them in pools and slow-moving waters. Larvae penetrate the skin usually in the feet or legs, invade veins and transform into adult male and female worms. Females deposit eggs in tissues, preferentially in the bowel and bladder where they cross the mucosa and are eliminated in stools and urine.

In humans, worms cause three different types of injury:

(i) granulomatous inflammation;
(ii) vessel obstruction;
(iii immune assault.

Inflammation is a local reaction evoked by parasites in tissues where they are trapped, mainly in the liver, heart and bladder, with a tropism that depends on the species, *S. Mansoni* and *S. Japonicum* in liver, *S. Hematobium* in urinary apparatus. Flukes invade vessels, e.g. mesenteric and outer bladder plexus and cause obstruction and inflammation. Finally, antibodies can form immune complexes that target the kidneys where they reproduce different forms of proliferative glomerulonephritis.

BALKAN NEPHROPATHY

Until the last decade of the last century, Balkan nephropathy has been a very localized disease occurring in people of small rural communities spread in the Balkan region. The disease was endemic and the probability for a physician not living in the region to meet a case was close to zero. In fact, the region was economically underdeveloped and people were restrained until democracy, national autonomy and admission to the European Union made it possible for Balkan people to travel and migrate.

Now meeting Balkan citizens in Western countries is not rare. Consider, for example, that Rumanians are the largest foreign community resident in Italy, around 1.2 million people. Consequently, one has to include Balkan nephropathy as the possible cause of a salt-losing disease in people native from that geographic area. A requisite for developing the disease, however, is having lived in the Balkans for at least 10-15 years, for its cause is toxicity of food containing Aristolochia products, a herb contaminating wheat cultivations.

The symptoms are those of a chronic salt-losing nephropathy (polyuria, hyponatremia, hypokalemia) slowly progressing to renal failure. In contrast with other salt-losing diseases blood pressure is high, probably because of a vasoconstriction caused by correct by the toxic herb.

REFERENCES

1. M. Florian, E.Wagenhner, E. Truls, J. Bjerklund, Z. Tandogdu: Epidemiology, definition and treatment of complicated urinary tract infections. *Nature Reviews Nephrology*, August 25, 2020. https://doi.org/10.1038/s415-020-0362-4
2. S.A. Howles, R.V. Thakker: Renal calculi. *Nature Reviews Nephrology*, June 12 2020 https://doi.org/10.1038/s415-020-0332-x